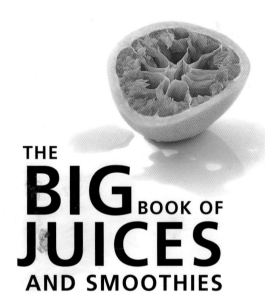

THE
BIG BOOK OF
JUICES
AND SMOOTHIES

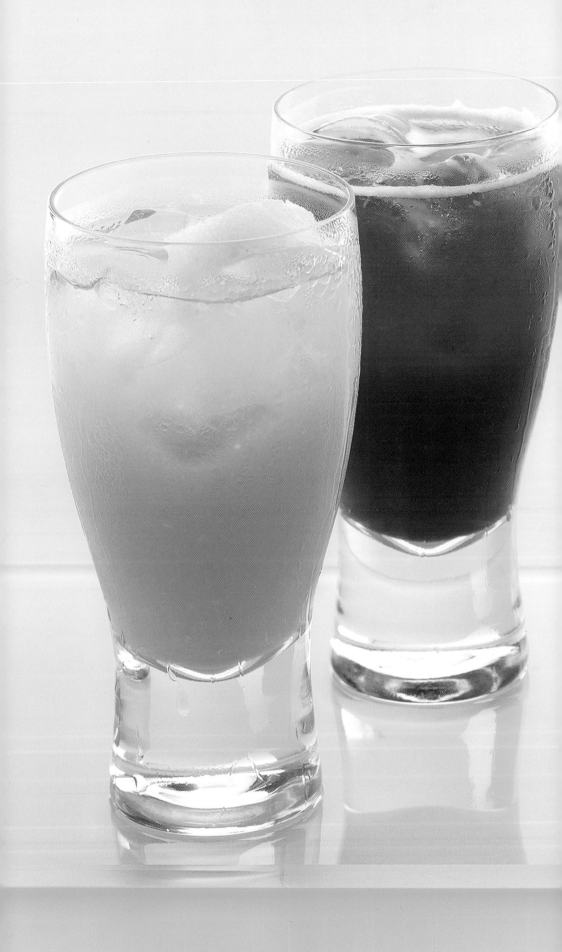

NATALIE SAVONA

THE BIG BOOK OF JUICES AND SMOOTHIES

365 NATURAL BLENDS FOR HEALTH AND VITALITY EVERY DAY

DUNCAN BAIRD PUBLISHERS

LONDON

The Big Book of Juices and Smoothies
Natalie Savona

First published in the United Kingdom
and Ireland in 2003 by
Duncan Baird Publishers Ltd
Sixth Floor, Castle House
75–76 Wells Street
London W1T 3QH

Conceived, created and designed by
Duncan Baird Publishers

Managing Editor: Judy Barratt
Editor: Rebecca Miles
Managing Designer: Manisha Patel
Designer: Allan Sommerville
Commissioned Photography: William Lingwood
Stylists: David Morgan (food) and
          Helen Trent

Juicer supplied by Theolife Ltd: Samson 6 in 1
Multipurpose Juice Extractor GB9001
www.samsonjuicer.co.uk

Cataloguing-in-publication data available from
the publisher.

10 9 8 7 6 5 4 3 2

ISBN: 1-904292-41-0

Typeset in Frutiger and Apollo MT
Colour reproduction by Scanhouse, Malaysia
Printed by Imago, China

Publisher's Note: None of the information
in this book is meant as a substitute for
professional medical advice. If you are in
any doubt as to the suitability of any of the
therapeutic methods or recipes given in this
book, consult your doctor.

Follow either the imperial or the metric
measurements when making the recipes.
The measurements are not interchangeable.

Author's acknowledgments
Thank you ... to nutritionist Jane Windsor-
Smith for her consultation work on the recipe
properties; to Judy Barratt, Becky Miles,
Manisha Patel and Allan Sommerville at DBP
for producing this beautiful book; to my
parents for giving me, among everything else,
one of the best juicers money can buy; to
Amanda Bluglass for being my juicing buddy
and so much more.

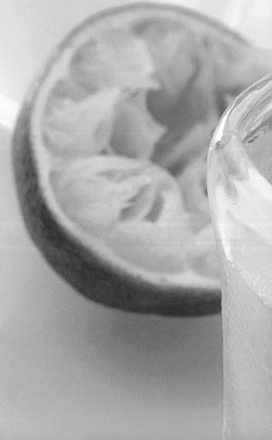

contents

introduction

The mouthwatering tang of freshly squeezed orange juice straight from squeezer to mouth within minutes – my early experiences of fresh juice was, as for most of us, from this staple citrus fruit. My first venture into the more alien world of vegetable juices came on a beach in Thailand – a large glass of frothy, deep orange carrot juice. This sublime taste in an exotic location marked the beginning of a culinary adventure.

First, using a basic, modestly-priced juicer salvaged from the depths of my parents' kitchen, I turned out concoctions of almost anything I had in the fruit bowl or refrigerator. As I became bolder, I requested an expensive, high-powered juicer as a present a few years ago and haven't looked back since.

The overriding selling point for all juices and smoothies is that they attain the magical quality, so elusive in so much of what we eat and drink today, of tasting sensational *and* being supremely good for you. Raw fruit and vegetables are laden with vitamins, minerals, enzymes and other ingredients that give us a boost in energy, help ward off illness and keep our bodies' cleansing processes working optimally.

Once you have developed the habit of making your own fresh juice combinations each morning, nothing else will do. I wager you will become so convinced that you would no sooner go without your daily juice than without brushing your teeth. Ahead of you are recipes for more juices and smoothies than you could ever ask for, not to mention a selection of frozen drinks and some refreshing teas. My breakfast is regularly

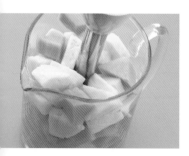 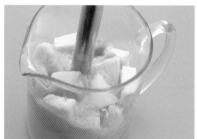 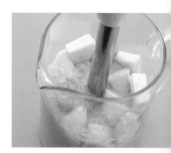

fresh, home-made juice and a creamy smoothie. You really couldn't get a much better start to the day.

how to use this book

This book provides you with 365 recipes to guide and inspire you to begin a daily juicing habit. It is organized into chapters of juices, smoothies and quenchers, each with its own coloured thumb tab for quick and easy reference. In addition, the tabs in chapters 2 and 3 ("making juices" and "making smoothies") show different fruit and vegetable icons denoting the prime ingredient around which a group of recipes is based. For example, a pear on a blue (juice) tab indicates a page of pear-based juice recipes, and a mango on a pink (smoothie) tab indicates mango-based smoothie recipes. In turn, these icons are used on yellow tabs in the ingredients lists in chapter 1. This handy tabbing system will allow you to choose recipes with ease, according to preference or what is in your refrigerator.

For further information on their specific health benefits, the recipes also list the main vitamins, minerals and other key nutrients in each drink. In addition, each recipe has a star-rating system giving the drink marks out of five for its energy-boosting, detoxing and immunity-boosting properties, and its benefits to the digestive system and the skin. At the end of the book, there is a nutrient chart providing further information on vitamins and minerals, and an ailments chart with suggested juices and smoothies to drink to help combat a range of common illnesses.

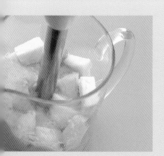 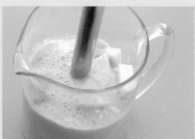 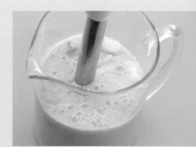

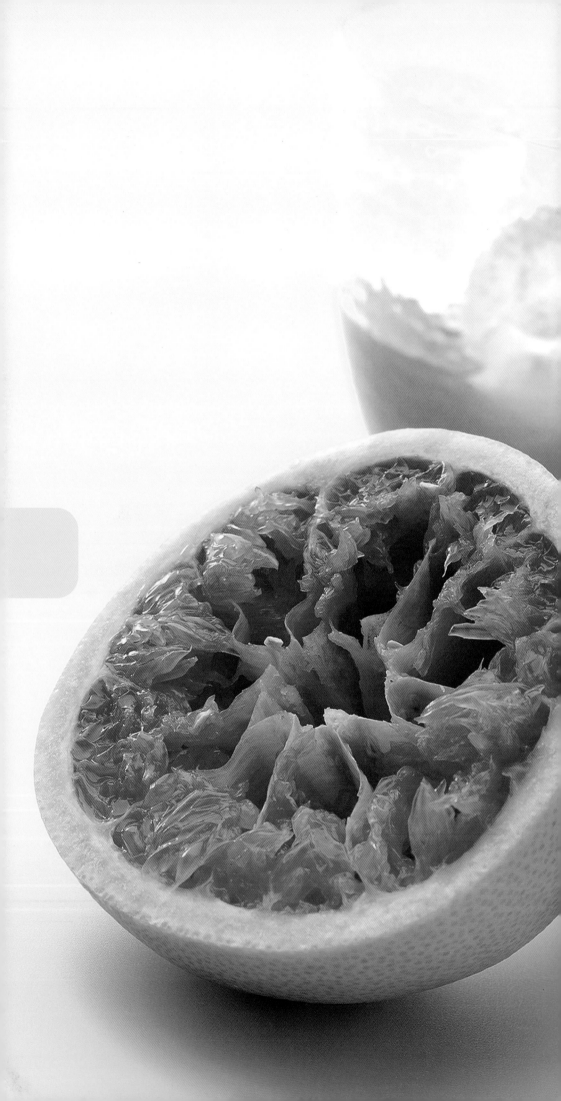

juicing
basics

chapter 1

You're sold on the idea that juicing is a good thing: you know that fresh juices are not only delicious but also packed with healthy ingredients. But before you go rushing out to buy a state-of-the-art juicer, take some time to absorb the advice presented in this chapter. This will help you get the most out of your juicing.

Over the following pages we look at the different kinds of juice drinks you can make and offer some suggestions on the basic kit you'll need. We explore why juices really are so good for you – we examine the many benefits of drinking juice daily and reveal how the body uses this direct source of nutrients for optimum health. We discover that there are few fruit and vegetables that cannot be consumed in the form of a nutritious drink, and learn how best to choose and prepare them. Finally, we look at some of the optional extras, such as flaxseeds and wheatgerm, that can add a healthy bonus to your glass.

why juice?

First of all, let us not forget that one of the most important aspects of anything we eat or drink is pleasure. Savouring a home-made, fresh juice is, for anyone who has tried it, an immensely pleasurable experience. Not only does it taste truly delicious, it also invigorates your body and mind, and gives the added satisfaction of having created it yourself.

Following on from the pleasure principle comes the effect that food and drink has on our body and mind. Raw, fresh juice is probably one of the most health-affirming, rejuvenating substances we can take. Drinking a fresh juice provides the body with nutrients on a superhighway – it's a fast delivery of vitamins, minerals, enzymes, carbohydrates, chlorophyll and countless other phytonutrients (nutrients derived from plants), which increasingly are being shown to boost health. And all of this contained in pure, fresh water. These natural blends of nutrients work together to enhance immunity, protecting us from not just colds and coughs but cancer and cardiovascular disease. Juices are powerhouses of antioxidants – nutrients such as vitamins A, C and E that fight oxidants (sometimes called free radicals) in our bodies which contribute to cancer, heart disease and aging. Other substances present in a juice, such as green chlorophyll, are particularly cleansing.

Even the least health-conscious person is now aware that we are supposed to have at least five servings of fruit and vegetables a day. Officially, a glass of juice counts a single portion, although immediately I'd say that a fresh, unadulterated, home-made juice, drunk straight from the jug, easily rates higher than your average shop-bought juice. A fresh juice also delivers the nutrients straight into your body within minutes, as it does not need to be digested in the way that fruit and vegetables do. And, given that some of your fruit, and probably all of your vegetables, are eaten at the same time as other foods, they are digested pretty slowly, and perhaps not too efficiently, so the nutrients may not be well absorbed.

So, in drinking your daily juice, you are not only fuelling yourself with energy, but you are also supporting your body's natural cleansing processes and helping stave off all manner of diseases. A home-made juice stands in a league of its own compared with off-the-shelf processed juices, not to mention coffee, tea, cordials, fizzy and so-called "energy" drinks, and is simply the best liquid refreshment that a body can have.

juice or smoothie?

So, what is the difference? It's really a question of semantics – you can call your juice drinks what you like but for the sake of clarity, I have chosen to make a distinction. Simply, a juice is a drink made using a special juice extractor or citrus press and a smoothie is a drink made by mixing whole ingredients into a pulp in a blender. This book divides smoothies into two basic categories – fruity and creamy – where a creamy smoothie has a richer, creamier texture owing to the addition of yogurt to the mix. Some further variations on the smoothie theme appear in Chapter 4, Making Quenchers. Here, frozen fruit, ice and sparkling water are added for an extra-chilled, refreshing taste.

Now that we've got the semantics clear, there is actually a great deal of difference in the consistency and properties of the end products. With a juice you are getting just that – the juice from the fruit or vegetable as it is pushed through the extractor or press and the fibre is left behind. Because a smoothie is made by simply blending the fruit to a pulp, you get the whole fruit, including the fibre, merely in a different form. A smoothie can be breakfast in itself; a juice may be just the first course.

There are particular benefits associated with both the juice and the smoothie group of drinks. Juices provide nutrients at top speed – our bodies absorb their goodness with maximum efficiency, unhindered by any need to break down and digest bulkier foodstuffs. The lack of any fibre (left behind in the juicing process) means that our bodies can assimilate the nutrients from a juice in a matter of minutes rather than hours.

This is a sure-fire way of getting the most out of the vitamins, minerals, enzymes, cleansing elements and other nutritional goodness from a fruit or vegetable. After drinking a fresh juice, you feel invigorated almost immediately. By doing this daily, you provide your body with a high dose of naturally derived nutrients that boosts your health and helps keep you well-protected against toxins and disease.

Unlike juices, smoothies contain a good amount of fibre, something that is an important nutrient in itself. Indeed, fibre is an essential and all-too-often lacking ingredient in our diets. Not only does it help keep our guts moving, but it also helps them to keep healthy and to maintain the right levels of good bacteria. In addition to this, any drink using yogurt or milk, such as our creamy smoothies, becomes an important source of protein, another essential in a healthy diet.

getting ready

equipment

To make a variety of the recipes from this book, you will need a juice extractor, a citrus press and a blender. All of the juice recipes can be made using a juice extractor alone, although citrus fruits are best squeezed on a proper citrus press; they tend to clog up a juicer and leave behind a lot of their precious juice. For the purposes of this book, when I say "juice" a piece of fruit, I mean put it into an electric juicer, and when I say "squeeze" a fruit, I mean extract its juice by squeezing it on a citrus press.

When choosing your first juicer, buy one one at the lower end of the price range which will give you a perfectly good introduction to the joy of juicing. Most juicers are what are called "centrifugal extractors", which means they grate the fruit and quickly spin it out toward a mesh which catches the pulp and sends the juice down into a jug. This can make quite a mess in the machine and I suggest cleaning it immediately, before you've even allowed yourself a sip of the end product. It really doesn't take more than a couple of minutes.

Once you are converted to the delights and blessings of daily juicing, you may want to invest in one of the more expensive machines. Like with most things in life, you tend to get what you pay for – the more expensive juicers are likely to have a hardier motor and extract more juice per piece of fruit.

Citrus presses can be bought for a reasonable price in most kitchen accessory shops or department stores. They usually take the form of a stainless steel structure around which you squeeze halved fruit, although electric ones are also available.

The essential piece of smoothie kit is a blender. Most kitchens have one, albeit maybe little-used, but, again, you can buy one quite cheaply and it can soon become a smoothie-making machine creating breakfast or a refreshing drink in a flash.

storing juices and smoothies

In my book, there really is no such thing as storing a juice or smoothie – you can't beat drinking them the moment you've made them. However, you may like to take them out to work or on a picnic. In that case, the best way to store them is to put a teaspoon of vitamin C powder or a squeeze of lemon juice in the bottom of the jug attached to the juicer. The vitamin C acts as an antioxidant, preventing the juice from turning brown. The same goes for smoothies. Also, keep the drinks covered and cool – in a sealed container in the refrigerator, or in a thermos flask.

the ingredients

choosing the best

Where possible, always choose fresh, local, organic produce that is in season. Organic fruits and vegetables provide you with all the goodness you need and none of the agrochemicals you don't. Also, buying locally supports your local economy and avoids adding to the economic and environmental costs of long-distance transport and storage of goods. (That said, you sometimes can't beat a delicious tropical mango or pineapple that has come all the way from India or Thailand!)

The following pages list information and preparation details for the fruits and vegetables used in the recipes (the foods follow the order of first appearance in the book). They are listed individually or in groups according to the batches of recipes within each chapter, and given a pictorial tab for easy reference.

fruits

Apple — The best apples for juices and smoothies are sharp, crisp ones such as Granny Smith, Braeburn, Egremont Russet or Discovery. Apples make a fantastic base juice and are laden with health properties from their vitamin, mineral, malic acid and fibre content. They are not only detoxifying but also good for lowering cholesterol, aiding digestion and improving the condition of the skin. *Preparation: Wash well. For juicing, simply remove stalk and cut into pieces small enough to fit through your juicer. For smoothies, core and chop.*

Grapefruit — The sharp flavour of even the sweetest grapefruit is remarkably refreshing. White, pink, red is the order of increasing sweetness. Like all citrus fruits, grapefruits are packed with vitamin C, so good for immunity. The pith contains the bioflavonoids (powerful antioxidants which work alongside vitamin C), so don't peel that off when juicing grapefruits. However, squeezing the fruit using a citrus press actually produces more juice, but you lose the bioflavanoids. *Preparation: If juicing, peel and cut to fit. If squeezing, cut in half.*

Orange — The classic fruit juice, and of course the best way to get the most out of the fruit is to cut into quarters, suck out the juice and nibble the flesh from the skin. However, you simply can't beat fresh, home-made orange juice. Oranges, with their high vitamin C and bioflavonoid content are the famous immune-booster, but they are also rich in minerals and very cleansing. You get the most juice by squeezing them, but juicing means you also benefit from the bioflavonoids in the pith. *Preparation: If juicing, peel and chop into chunks. If squeezing, cut in half.*

Raspberry — Plump, summer raspberries may warrant popping into the mouth as is, but they do make a wonderful addition to a juice or blended drink. Like all berries, they are a rich source of nutrients, especially antioxidants. (This tab is used in the juice chapter only.) *Preparation: Wash well. Pick out any that are mouldy or still attached to the hulls.*

Peach, **nectarine** and **apricot** are from the same botanical family and their drinks appear in the book under the same pictorial tab.

Peach — Good peaches yield a fantastic, rich nectar, ideal for blended drinks. Because of their high beta-carotene content, peaches help protect against lung, skin and digestive problems. With countless varieties of colour, it's best to choose a peach by its tenderness and its smell. A good peach will yield to a gentle squeeze and have a sweet scent, but an under-ripe specimen will be hard and barely smell of anything. *Preparation: Wash well. Halve, remove stone and chop into chunks.*

Nectarine — The bald relative of peaches, good nectarines also burst with an orange, sweet nectar. They are a rich source of beta-carotene, as well as vitamin C and a spectrum of minerals. Use only when they are tender to a gentle squeeze in the palm. *Preparation: Wash well. Halve, remove stone and chop into chunks.*

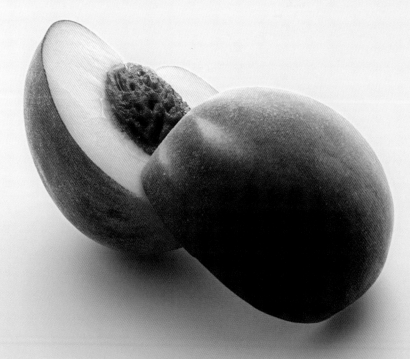

Apricot — You're likely to get sweeter apricots in mid- and late-summer rather than earlier in the year. Choose them slightly soft to the touch and smelling sweet as they're unlikely to ripen further. Also, the riper they are, the higher their beta-carotene content. As a winter alternative soaked, dried apricots make a delicious, sweet addition to a smoothie. *Preparation (fresh apricots): Wash well. Halve and remove stone.*

Cherry — A luxury inasmuch as you need time and patience to yield a decent quantity of stoned, fresh fruit. But you will be grateful not only for the intense flavour of the juice: cherries contain rich antioxidant nutrients as well as highly alkaline properties, particularly good for arthritis and gout. *Preparation: Wash well. Slice in half and prise out the stone or use an olive stoner.*

Pear — As with many fruits, I hesitate to hand ripe Williams pears to my juicer rather than eat them straight up. While a juicy, ripe pear is best for blending, use a slightly under-ripe pear for juicing, even Comice or Conference varieties, and you will get a surprisingly thick yield. Similar to apples, pears are very cleansing and full of a range of vitamins, minerals and fibre. *Preparation: Wash well. For juicing, simply remove stalk and cut into pieces small enough to fit through your juicer. For smoothies, core and chop.*

Pineapple — The delicious flesh of the pineapple is a perfect juice or smoothie ingredient. It is rich in a range of vitamins and minerals, but is particularly known for an alkaline substance called bromelain, which aids digestion and is linked to a reduction of inflammation in arthritis and other inflammatory disorders. Choose a pineapple that is a deep, yellow colour and gives off a sweet scent from the bottom. *Preparation: Chop off the top and bottom of the fruit, and slice down the sides to remove the skin. If blending, remove any remaining eyes (there's no need if you are juicing).*

Banana — Completely unjuiceable, but a wonderful staple for blended drinks, turning a smoothie into a meal in itself. As with most fruit the riper the banana, the richer the flavour, and they're even good in a drink when they are past their eating best. A banana is a nutritional powerhouse – full of fibre, vitamins and minerals, as well as carbohydrates which are a key source of energy. *Preparation: Peel and break or slice into pieces.*

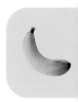

Mango — Mangoes, one of nature's most sumptuous fruits, come in a variety of colours and sizes, although my favourite are the amber Alfonse variety from India (usually available in late spring). Otherwise, choose your mango carefully to avoid disappointment: look out for one that yields slightly to the thumb and smells sweet (don't be fooled by the colour, as some green mangoes are perfectly ripe). Mangoes are extremely rich in beta-carotene, as well as minerals such as magnesium. *Preparation: Peel and slice flesh away from the stone. (Then chew and suck it unashamedly!)*

Papaya — One of the Tropics' wonderfoods, the papaya (or paw paw) is packed with beta-carotene, enzymes that help digestion, vitamin C and fibre. It comes in several varieties, although the most common is the more squat, pear-shaped type. Papayas are ripe when they are fully amber in colour and yield to gentle pressure. *Preparation: Peel, remove seeds, and slice into chunks.*

Drinks based on a variety of **berries** (including some recipes containing raspberries and strawberries) appear under this pictorial tab in the smoothie chapter.

> **Blackberry** — One of the few fruits that we can continue to pick wild. All the scratches are worth the effort for a pile of freshly picked, plump blackberries. Otherwise, nip down to the local green-grocer store. Blackberries are rich in antioxidants, particularly vitamin C. *Preparation: Wash well. Discard any berries that are mouldy or still attached to the hulls.*

Blackcurrant — Sharp but not sour, perfectly ripe blackcurrants add a strong flavour to any drink. They are an extremely rich source of vitamin C and other antioxidant nutrients. Crunch their seeds well in a blended drink as they contain healthy essential fats. *Preparation: Wash well. Remove any stalks and discard any berries that are mouldy.*

Blueberry — Small in size, big in flavour and goodness, blueberries are laden with antioxidant nutrients such as vitamins A and C, as well as bioflavonoids. They yield a rich, sweet flavour and give a blended drink blue specks. The berries are good for overcoming bladder problems, as well as boosting immunity and protecting the eyes and blood vessels. *Preparation: Wash well. Remove any stalks and discard any berries that are mouldy.*

Cranberry — Cranberries are excellent therapy for male and female urinary-tract problems but only in their pure, unsweetened form – the sweeteners often present in commercial drinks can aggravate such conditions. Because they are rather tart, cranberries are best mixed with other fruits. Like all berries, they are rich in a range of antioxidant nutrients. *Preparation: Wash well. Remove any stalks and discard any berries that are spoiled.*

Drinks using fruits belonging to the **melon** family are listed under this pictorial tab (they appear only in chapter three).

Cantaloupe/Honeydew — These are the most widely available varieties of melon. The orange-fleshed cantaloupe is particularly high in beta-carotene, but both kinds are rich in a range of vital nutrients, especially vitamin C. They have diuretic properties, meaning that they help eliminate excess fluid from the body. Choose melons that are firm, but yield slightly to pressing and that smell sweet. *Preparation: Halve, slice and cut the flesh away from the rind. Chop into chunks.*

Watermelon — Loaded with water and minerals, watermelon is one of the easiest healthfoods to digest.

Its redness indicates its high levels of beta-carotene, although it is also rich in minerals, especially potassium, and is a great cleanser. Blitz the seeds in the blender too, for extra zinc and vitamin E. Choose a watermelon that feels heavy for its size and makes a hollow sound when tapped. *Preparation: Cut out a wedge from the whole fruit and cut the flesh away from the rind. Chop to fit.*

Strawberry — Probably the most abundant and popular berry in the West, the strawberry is also one of the richest food sources of vitamin C. It is also abundant in a range of beneficial minerals, especially calcium which is good for bones and teeth. *Preparation: Wash well and, if blending, remove hulls (no need if juicing).*

The following fruits also appear in the recipes, but not as base ingredients. However, it is worth noting their nutritional value.

Date — Clearly not for juicing, but dates provide a rich, natural sweetness to a smoothie and load it with energy from the sugar. They're also a useful source of vitamin C. The best are the large, soft, sticky Medjool variety. *Preparation: Wash, halve and remove the pits.*

Grape — The grape is a very cleansing, alkaline, nutritious fruit, which is why grape-juice diets have been used for many years to heal chronic illnesses. The seedless varieties of either green or red grapes should be used for drinks, although red grapes are richer in antioxidants, notably those which can help reduce the threat of heart disease. *Preparation: Wash well.*

Guava — Not easy to get hold of, but if you do come across some guavas, they make fantastic, tropical additions to a drink. Choose fruits with a green-yellow skin – the fruit and the juice will be white to pink. Many stores sell guava nectar, but be sure to buy unsweetened brands. *Preparation: Peel, halve, remove seeds and chop into chunks.*

Kiwi — The brown, hairy exterior of the kiwi fruit belies its beautiful green interior with magically patterned black seeds. One of the richest sources of vitamin C, kiwis are also laden with beneficial minerals, especially potassium. Unfortunately, like much fresh produce these days, they are usually picked too early, but will ripen at home – just make sure they don't get too soft and develop a sweet acetone flavour. *Preparation: Peel and chop into chunks.*

Lemon — Too tart to ever be drunk neat, lemon juice is perfect for toning down the sweetness or saltiness of other juices, or even for being diluted with hot or cold water. Rich in vitamin C and bioflavonoids (mainly in the pith), lemons are also high in a range of minerals and are a particularly good source of potassium. To extract the maximum amount of juice, choose lemons that are heavy given their size and feel slightly soft. *Preparation: If juicing, peel and chop into chunks. If squeezing, cut in half.*

Lime — The smaller, green relative of lemons, limes have similar health properties and add a wonderful tropical tang to juices. *Preparation: If juicing, peel and chop into chunks. If squeezing, cut in half.*

Passion fruit — The uglier and wrinklier the passion fruit, the more likely it is to be full and juicy. Each fruit should have orange flesh, grey seeds and a pink inner lining. Passion fruit is a good source of vitamin C and has a richly perfumed flavour that stands out in almost any drink. *Preparation: Cut in half and scoop out flesh.*

Tangerine — Similar to the orange, but sweeter and with a far looser skin, any one of the tangerine/clementine family are a refreshing, milder alternative to this staple juice. Although you get the most juice by squeezing tangerines, putting them through a juicer will give you bioflavonoids in the pith. *Preparation: If juicing, peel and chop into chunks. If squeezing, cut in half.*

vegetables

There are few vegetable juices, other than carrot, that are drinkable neat: most are simply not palatable enough. They are also generally too strong and should be diluted with other juices.

Carrot — The sweetest and best-tasting of vegetable juices, carrots are packed with vitamins and minerals, not least the antioxidant beta-carotene. The carrot's overall nutrient value makes it an immune-boosting, skin-clearing, digestion-supporting drink. *Preparation: Scrub well, top and tail and cut to fit.*

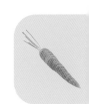

Cucumber — Cucumber juice is surprisingly flavourful, given the bland nature of the vegetable. Because of its mineral balance and high water content, cucumber is one of the best, natural diuretics known. Choose firm, dark cucumbers. *Preparation: Wash well and chop to fit.*

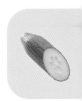

Green vegetable juice drinks are listed under this pictorial tab which can be found in chapter two.

Watercress — Watercress is a very powerful cleanser owing to its high chlorophyll and sulphur contents. It is good for digestion, the skin, the circulation and the bladder, and is an exceptional, all-round juice. Because it is so potent, watercress is best well-diluted with other juices. Choose only green leaves, discarding any that have started to go yellow. *Preparation: Wash well.*

Broccoli — With even more vitamin C than oranges (pound for pound), broccoli is loaded with important antioxidant and cleansing nutrients, some of which have been shown to protect against cancer. Choose compact, green heads for the freshest, most nutritious juice. *Preparation: Wash well and cut to fit your juicer.*

Cabbage — Although on its own it is not particularly palatable as a juice, cabbage is worth slipping into other juices for its far-reaching health properties. Like other members of its family (broccoli, kale and so on), cabbage is full of vitamins, minerals and anti-cancer nutrients. It is also soothing for stomach problems, including ulcers. *Preparation: Remove outer leaves and cut off pieces to fit.*

Kale — One of nature's wonderfoods, kale is loaded with vitamins (especially A and C) and minerals as well as anti-cancer nutrients. As such it is a very cleansing, immune-boosting, skin-healing, bone-building, generally excellent all-round health bonanza. *Preparation: Wash well.*

Lettuce — Choose the darker varieties, which tend to be richer in all minerals and vitamins. Lettuce is cleansing because of the combination of nutrients and high water content, but it is also known for its sedative properties and is best added to juices as a relaxant or sleep aid. *Preparation: Wash leaves well.*

Parsley — Parsley is one of the top ingredients in the health stakes. Its dark green colour comes from its rich chlorophyll content, which makes it highly cleansing. Parsley is also good for aiding digestion and for generally providing the body with a stack of minerals and vitamins. *Preparation: Wash well.*

Spinach — Exceptionally rich in vitamin C, beta-carotene and iron, spinach is also highly cleansing and is laden with health-boosting, regenerative properties. These tone the digestive system, the liver and the circulation. However, it is high in oxalic acid, which interferes with calcium absorption, so spinach juice should not be drunk in large quantities. Choose small, bright green leaves. *Preparation: Wash well.*

Root vegetable juice drinks (other than the carrot) can be found under this pictorial tab in chapter two.

Beet (beetroot) — The wonderful juice of beet has a distinctly "soily" taste to it. This earthiness gives a hint of the very rich mineral and vitamin content, and as such, beet is one of the most cleansing, blood-boosting, tonic-like juices there is. Juice the greens too, if you can get hold of them, as they add an even greater health dimension. *Preparation: Top and tail, scrub well and cut to fit.*

Parsnip — This white relative of the carrot provides a sweet, earthy touch to a juice, as well as an all-round dose of minerals and vitamins for the body. Parsnip is rich in the trace elements sulphur and silicon, good for healthy hair, skin and nails. *Preparation: Scrub well, top and tail and cut to fit.*

Sweet potato — Not related to the potato, sweet potatoes are generally easier to digest and higher in fibre than their namesakes. They are also a rich source of beta-carotene. Sweet potatoes are soothing to the digestive tract, cleansing, and have an alkalizing effect on the body. *Preparation: Scrub well and cut to fit.*

Tomato — Although strictly speaking a fruit, the tomato is commonly classed as a vegetable as it has a savoury rather than a sweet taste. Tomatoes taste quite acidic, but, in fact, have a soothing effect on the body. They offer nutrients which can ease problems with digestion, the liver and the skin. Tomatoes also contain lycopene, an antioxidant shown to help prostate problems. *Preparation: Wash well and slice to fit.*

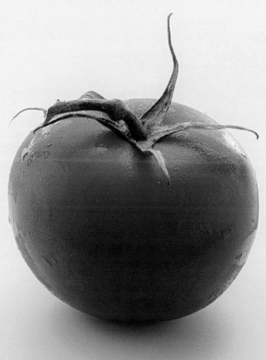

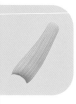

Celery — A refreshing, salty juice, celery complements other vegetable juice flavours by cutting through some of the richer, sweeter tastes. Celery is a very cleansing, soothing juice, with diuretic properties (helping to rid the body of excess water). Choose greener stems, not those that are wilting or bendy. Juice the whole stick, including the leaves. *Preparation: Scrub well.*

Other ingredients used in some of the recipes in this book include the following:

> **Bell Peppers** — Also called peppers or capsicum, red, green and yellow bell peppers add a sweet flavour to juice and are an excellent source of antioxidants, particularly vitamin C and beta-carotene. *Preparation: Wash well and slice.*
>
> **Ginger** — An age-old natural remedy, the root of the ginger plant helps improve digestion and circulation, and relieves nausea, bloating, colds, sore throats and inflammation of any sort. *Preparation: Wash well, peel if shrivelled and slice.*
>
> **Mint** — This aromatic herb is a refreshing, soothing addition to a drink. It helps to enhance digestion and calm the digestive tract, quell nausea and relieve cramps. The menthol in mint can also soothe congestion in the respiratory tract. Choose fresh, deep green leaves. *Preparation: Wash well.*

healthy additives

You can enhance the health properties of your juice or smoothie even further by adding certain vitamin and mineral supplements, and other health-enhancing foods. Some of the additives are best blended with smoothies only, as they don't mix well in a pure, liquid juice.

additives for juices or smoothies

Vitamin and mineral drops/powder — Some companies make excellent vitamins and minerals in the form of liquid drops or powders. Adding them to your daily juice or smoothie is a good way of taking them, especially for children.

Herbal drops — If you take herbal medicines, such as echinacea or a blend from your herbalist, mixing them with a juice may be a more palatable option. (Check with your herbalist whether or not mixing with just water may be better.)

Spirulina/Barleygrass/Wheatgrass powder — Dense forms of nutrients especially rich in cleansing chlorophyll, these three are nature's wonderfoods in a green powder. If you're mixing one with juice, best to shake it with a little juice in a jar before blending it with the rest.

smoothie-only additives

Wheatgerm — Most of the goodness in a grain of wheat is found in the germ – a great additive to smoothies for an extra boost of vitamins and minerals, particularly vitamins B and E.

Flaxseeds — Also known as linseeds, one of the richest vegetarian sources of essential fatty acids, as well as vitamins and minerals.

Pumpkin/sunflower seeds — These not only give smoothies a nutty, crunchy taste and texture, but also increase their vitamin, mineral and essential fatty acid content.

Cold-pressed seed oils — Far from the usual commercial varieties, cold-pressed oils, such as from sunflower or pumpkin seeds, offer unadulterated sources of essential fatty acids.

Tahini — This creamed sesame seed paste adds a distinctive flavour to any smoothie, as well as boosting its nutrient content.

Blackstrap molasses — Derived from the whole cane from which sugar is extracted, syrupy sweet molasses is laden with minerals (particularly iron and calcium) and B-vitamins.

Lecithin — Part of every cell of the body, lecithin is particularly important for the digestion of fats and for healthy nerve and brain cells. Add it to your smoothie in powder form.

Brewer's yeast — This is one of the best sources of B-vitamins available, and also contains a host of vital minerals.

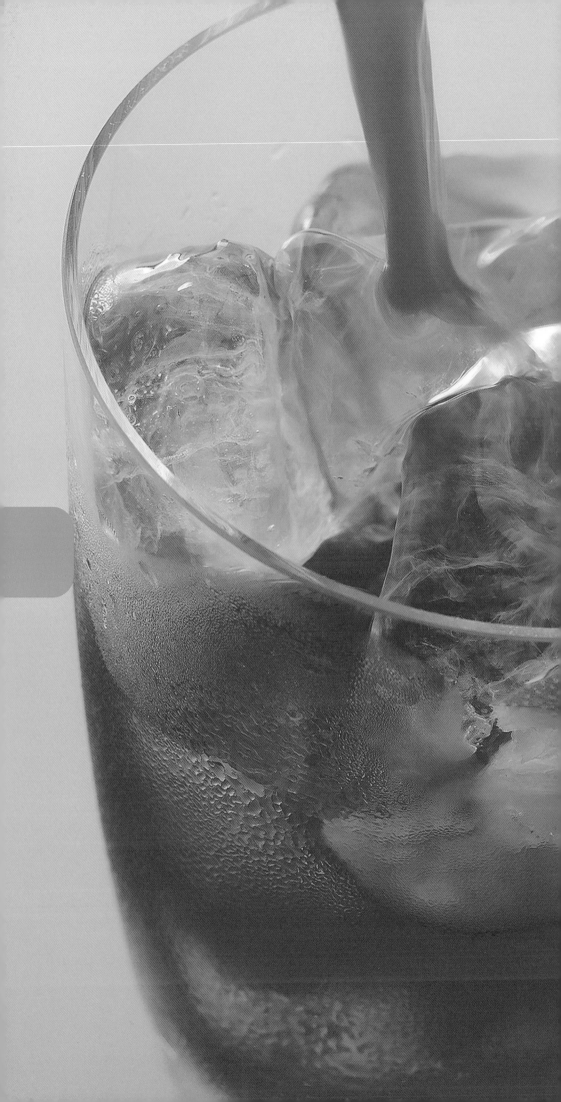

making
juices
chapter 2

Once you start on the adventure of making a fresh juice every day, you will be hooked. By now you are aware of the delights and benefits of pressing your own juice and here's where the actual process begins. You've got the juicer (you may even have used it), what follows on the next pages are 220 blends to stimulate both your palate and your imagination.

We begin with juices based on fruits (blends 1–128), followed by juices based on vegetables (blends 129–220). Each recipe makes two portions unless otherwise stated. If you feel you'd like some guidance on which recipes to try first, you may like to experiment with The Basic Intro Week (see p.176) which will gently introduce you to the idea of blending different fruits and a few vegetables. Guidelines for preparing the ingredients are given on pages 14 to 24, so simply get them ready and juice away!

top tips

Below are a few reminders, and helpful hints, tips and suggestions to enable you to get the most from your juicing.

1   When selecting fruit to juice, choose pieces that are almost but not quite ripe, as these tend to yield the maximum amount of juice and the best taste from your juicer.

2   Avoid juicing fruits that are over-ripe or too soft as these generally do not pass well through a juicer.

3   Get into the habit of always washing your juicer immediately after use, when it is much easier to clean.

4   To get the most out of citrus fruits, extract the juice using a citrus press rather than a juicer.

5   While all fruit and veg must be washed well before use, avoid soaking them as this can weaken their nutrient content.

6   If you do peel your fruit or veg, do it as finely as possible so as to preserve as many of the vital nutrients as you can.

7   To prevent juices from going even slightly brown (that is oxidizing and damaging their nutrient content), drink them immediately or pour them into a jug containing a squeeze of lemon juice or a spoon of vitamin C powder.

8   Dilute your vegetable juices with a little water if you find them too strong-tasting. Always dilute vegetable juices for children.

9   If you find that your energy levels fluctuate throughout the day, emphasize vegetable juices, and dilute any fruit juices you do have with water. Fruit juices contain high levels of natural sugar which give an immediate energy boost but can be followed by a dip in your energy level.

10   Although you won't ever be stuck for recipes using this book, be experimental and create your own blends using whatever you have in the refrigerator and fruit bowl.

001 | eve's downfall

4 apples

I always have a sense that if you're going to make the effort to make a juice then make it interesting, but pure, freshly pressed apple juice is exquisite and you can't beat the home-made frothy, delicate green version. My favourite are Granny Smith or Egremont Russets but you could juice any type of apple you like.

NUTRIENTS

Beta-carotene, folic acid, vitamin C; calcium, magnesium, phosphorus, potassium, sulphur

ENERGY	★★★★★
DETOX	★★★★☆
IMMUNITY	★★☆☆☆
DIGESTION	★★★☆☆
SKIN	★★★☆☆

002 | apple basic

3 apples
2 carrots

Most of us can rustle up a few apples from the fruit bowl and carrots from the refrigerator. This delicious but simple combination is a good way to introduce carrot to your juice repertoire if you're not used to vegetable juices.

NUTRIENTS

Beta-carotene, folic acid, vitamin C; calcium, magnesium, phosphorus, potassium, sodium, sulphur

ENERGY	★★★★☆
DETOX	★★★★☆
IMMUNITY	★★☆☆☆
DIGESTION	★★☆☆☆
SKIN	★★★★☆

003 | ocean deep

4 apples
1 teaspoon spirulina

The combination of the pale green apple juice and dark green spirulina powder makes this power-packed juice look like the deep, green sea. Shake the spirulina with a little of the juice in a jar before mixing it with the rest.

NUTRIENTS

Beta-carotene, folic acid, vitamins B1, B2, B3, B5, B6 and C; calcium, magnesium, phosphorus, potassium, sulphur; protein, essential fatty acids

ENERGY	★★★★☆
DETOX	★★★★☆
IMMUNITY	★★★☆☆
DIGESTION	★★☆☆☆
SKIN	★★★★☆

004 | basic with a boost

3 apples
2 carrots
$\frac{1}{2}$ inch (1 cm) ginger root
1 teaspoon spirulina

The addition of spirulina sends the nutritious value of this juice onto another plane. Stir or shake in the spirulina powder after you have made the juice.

NUTRIENTS

Beta-carotene, folic acid, vitamin C; calcium, magnesium, phosphorus, potassium, sulphur; protein, essential fatty acids

ENERGY	★★★☆☆
DETOX	★★★★☆
IMMUNITY	★★★☆☆
DIGESTION	★★★☆☆
SKIN	★★★☆☆

005 | orchard blend

3 apples
1 pear

Made with classic orchard fruits, this sweet juice really makes you realize why apples and pears are the staples of a fruit bowl and not so boring after all.

NUTRIENTS

Beta-carotene, folic acid, vitamin C; calcium, magnesium, phosphorus, potassium, sulphur

ENERGY	★★★★☆
DETOX	★★☆☆☆
IMMUNITY	★★☆☆☆
DIGESTION	★★★☆☆
SKIN	★★★☆☆

006 | apple blush

3 apples
1 nectarine
8 strawberries

The delicate colour of this juice gives only the slightest indication of the sensational taste, especially if you use a tangy variety of apple such as Granny Smith combined with sweet, ripe strawberries and nectarines.

NUTRIENTS

Beta-carotene, biotin, folic acid, vitamin C; calcium, magnesium, phosphorus, potassium, sulphur

ENERGY	★★★★★
DETOX	★★☆☆☆
IMMUNITY	★★★☆☆
DIGESTION	★☆☆☆☆
SKIN	★★★★☆

007 | sweet 'n' savoury

3 apples
2 sticks celery

The saltiness of the celery nicely offsets the sweetness of the apples in this refreshing juice. It's a perfect thirst-quencher, especially if you use a sharp apple variety such as Granny Smith.

NUTRIENTS

Beta-carotene, folic acid, vitamin C; calcium, magnesium, manganese, phosphorus, potassium, sodium, sulphur

ENERGY	★★☆☆☆
DETOX	★★★☆☆
IMMUNITY	★☆☆☆☆
DIGESTION	★★★☆☆
SKIN	★★★☆☆

008 | sweet c

3 apples
2 guavas

This is one of the few recipes for which I suggest using a sweeter variety of apple, such as Cox, to offset the tangy guava, which is a phenomenally rich source of vitamin C.

NUTRIENTS

Beta-carotene, folic acid, vitamin B3, vitamin C; calcium, magnesium, phosphorus, potassium, sodium, sulphur

ENERGY	★★★★☆
DETOX	★★★☆☆
IMMUNITY	★★★★★
DIGESTION	★☆☆☆☆
SKIN	★★★★☆

009 | sweet c too

2 apples
2 oranges

You may think that oranges would completely overwhelm the delicate juice of the apples, but actually they really enhance it and make this drink a simple, refreshing start to the day. Remember that oranges are best juiced on a citrus press and added to the apple juice made in the extractor, although you can push peeled orange pieces through the juicer.

NUTRIENTS

Beta-carotene, folic acid, vitamin C; calcium, magnesium, phosphorus, potassium, sodium, sulphur

ENERGY	★★★★☆
DETOX	★★★☆☆
IMMUNITY	★★★★☆
DIGESTION	★☆☆☆☆
SKIN	★★★☆☆

010 | apple tropics

3 apples
$\frac{1}{2}$ pineapple
$\frac{1}{2}$ lime
$\frac{1}{2}$ passion fruit

An extra tang and taste of the tropics is evident in this apple recipe. It's best to stir the passion fruit into the juice once it's made, rather than passing it through the blender.

NUTRIENTS

Beta-carotene, folic acid, vitamin C; calcium, magnesium, manganese, phosphorus, potassium, sulphur

ENERGY	★★★★☆
DETOX	★★☆☆☆
IMMUNITY	★★★☆☆
DIGESTION	★★★★☆
SKIN	★★★☆☆

011 | citrus apples

3 apples
2 tangerines
$\frac{1}{2}$ lime

The more delicate flavour of tangerines (or clementines or other such fruits, rather than oranges) adds a subtle layer around the apple, while the lime gives it a great afterbite.

NUTRIENTS

Beta-carotene, folic acid, vitamin C; calcium, magnesium, phosphorus, potassium, sodium, sulphur

ENERGY	★★★☆☆
DETOX	★★☆☆☆
IMMUNITY	★★★★☆
DIGESTION	★☆☆☆☆
SKIN	★★★☆☆

012 | apple cleanser

2 apples
2 kale leaves
1 stick celery
$\frac{1}{3}$ long cucumber
$\frac{1}{2}$ beet (beetroot)

The fruitiness of the apples offsets the more challenging taste of the greens to produce this beautifully red detoxifying juice.

NUTRIENTS
Beta-carotene, folic acid, vitamin B3, vitamin C; calcium, iron, magnesium, manganese, phosphorus, potassium, sulphur

ENERGY	★★☆☆☆
DETOX	★★★★☆
IMMUNITY	★★★☆☆
DIGESTION	★★☆☆☆
SKIN	★★★☆☆

013 | winter crumble

2 apples
2 handfuls blackberries

I can't help but think of a hot pie or crumble when I make this juice. You could actually heat it up (but don't let it boil) after you've made it, for a warm drink on a cold night, but personally I like my juices cold.

NUTRIENTS
Beta-carotene, folic acid, vitamin B3, vitamin C; calcium, iron, magnesium, manganese, phosphorus, potassium, sodium, sulphur

ENERGY	★★★★★
DETOX	★★☆☆☆
IMMUNITY	★★★★☆
DIGESTION	★☆☆☆☆
SKIN	★★★★☆

014 | apple pie

4 apples
$\frac{1}{2}$ teaspoon ground cinnamon

It's quite hard to stir in the cinnamon powder – instead I suggest putting the juice in a jar and shaking it up to add the spicy kick.

NUTRIENTS

Beta-carotene, folic acid, vitamin B3,
vitamin C; calcium, magnesium,
phosphorus, potassium, sodium,
sulphur

ENERGY	★★★★☆
DETOX	★★★☆☆
IMMUNITY	★★☆☆☆
DIGESTION	★★★☆☆
SKIN	★★★☆☆

015 | apple blues

3 apples
2 good handfuls blueberries

If your blueberries are particularly sweet, choose a crisp, tangy apple such as Granny Smith; otherwise, use a sweeter type like Jonagold or Empire.

NUTRIENTS

Beta-carotene, biotin, folic acid,
vitamins B1, B2, B6, C and E; calcium,
chromium, magnesium, sodium

ENERGY	★★★★★
DETOX	★★★☆☆
IMMUNITY	★★★★☆
DIGESTION	★☆☆☆☆
SKIN	★★★★☆

016 | black orchard berry buster

3 apples
2 good handfuls dark berries such as blueberries,
    blackcurrants or blackberries

It may seem a waste to juice plump, sweet berries, but I can't resist it sometimes. In the winter you can throw a few canned berries into the juicer but it's not quite the same thing.

NUTRIENTS

Beta-carotene, folic acid,
vitamins B1, B2, B6, C and E; calcium,
chromium, magnesium, manganese,
phosphorus, potassium, sodium,
sulphur

ENERGY	★★★★★
DETOX	★★★☆☆
IMMUNITY	★★★★☆
DIGESTION	★☆☆☆☆
SKIN	★★★★☆

017 | pink orchard berry buster

3 apples
2 good handfuls red berries such as raspberries or
   strawberries

Another treat, using fresh, sweet berries in the summer to turn tangy apple
juice into a pastel thirst-quencher.

NUTRIENTS

Beta-carotene, biotin, folic acid,
vitamin C; calcium, magnesium,
manganese, phosphorus, potassium,
sodium, sulphur

ENERGY	★★★☆☆
DETOX	★☆☆☆☆
IMMUNITY	★★★★☆
DIGESTION	★☆☆☆☆
SKIN	★★★★☆

018 | double apple

2 apples
$\frac{1}{3}$ pineapple
1 small bunch fresh mint

Living in Bangkok, apples were a luxury, unlike the ubiquitous pineapple.
Unfortunately, it's completely the other way around in most other parts of
the world. Use sweeter apples such as Cox to match with the amazing juicy
tang of the pineapple, which is particularly helpful for digestion.

NUTRIENTS

Beta-carotene, folic acid, vitamin B3,
vitamin C; calcium, magnesium,
manganese, phosphorus, potassium,
sodium, sulphur

ENERGY	★★★☆☆
DETOX	★☆☆☆☆
IMMUNITY	★★★☆☆
DIGESTION	★★★★★
SKIN	★★☆☆☆

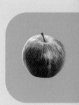

019 | waldorf salad

2 apples
2 sticks celery
1 dessertspoon (15 ml) cold-pressed hemp-seed oil

This one reminds me of a Waldorf salad, without the walnuts but with the
hemp-seed oil to give you a similar benefit of omega 3 fatty acids. The oil will
blend best if it's shaken with the juice in a jar.

NUTRIENTS

Beta-carotene, folic acid, vitamin C;
calcium, magnesium, manganese,
phosphorus, potassium, sodium,
sulphur; essential fatty acids

ENERGY	★★★★☆
DETOX	★★★☆☆
IMMUNITY	★★★☆☆
DIGESTION	★★★☆☆
SKIN	★★★☆☆

020 | bleeding apples

3 apples
½ beet (beetroot)

The colour of beet overtakes any other juice and gives it a deep,
earthy flavour. This recipe is a gentle introduction to the powerful
juice of this root vegetable. For heftier doses, see pp.95–6.

NUTRIENTS

Beta-carotene, folic acid, vitamin C;
calcium, magnesium, phosphorus,
potassium, sodium, sulphur

ENERGY	★★★★☆
DETOX	★★★★★
IMMUNITY	★★☆☆☆
DIGESTION	★★☆☆☆
SKIN	★★★☆☆

021 | apple tang

3 apples
1 grapefruit
1 lime

The sweetness of the apple – best to use a sweet variety – combines
well with the grapefruit and lime.

NUTRIENTS

Beta-carotene, folic acid, vitamin C;
calcium, magnesium, phosphorus,
potassium, sodium, sulphur

ENERGY	★★★★☆
DETOX	★★☆☆☆
IMMUNITY	★★★☆☆
DIGESTION	★☆☆☆☆
SKIN	★★★☆☆

022 | apple gone loupey

3 apples
2 thick slices of melon
1 small bunch fresh mint

To contrast with the sweetness of a ripe melon, it's best to use a sharper
apple variety such as Egremont Russet or Granny Smith.

NUTRIENTS

Beta-carotene, folic acid, vitamin C;
calcium, magnesium, phosphorus,
potassium, sodium, sulphur

ENERGY	★★★★★
DETOX	★★★☆☆
IMMUNITY	★★★☆☆
DIGESTION	★☆☆☆☆
SKIN	★★★★☆

023 | waterapple

3 apples
2 thick slices of watermelon
1 lime

I would usually use watermelon to make a fresh smoothie (see p.136), but this juice combination is irresistible. Use a sharp type of apple.

NUTRIENTS

Beta-carotene, folic acid, vitamin C; calcium, magnesium, phosphorus, potassium, sulphur

ENERGY	★★★★★
DETOX	★★★★☆
IMMUNITY	★★★☆☆
DIGESTION	★☆☆☆☆
SKIN	★★★★☆

024 | apple lullaby

2 apples
$\frac{1}{4}$ lettuce
$\frac{1}{2}$ lemon
(makes one glass of juice)

The lettuce is the key sleep-inducing ingredient in this juice. Best drunk just as you plan to hit the pillow. You can use any variety of lettuce.

NUTRIENTS

Beta-carotene, folic acid, vitamin C; calcium, magnesium, phosphorus, potassium, sulphur

ENERGY	★☆☆☆☆
DETOX	★★★☆☆
IMMUNITY	★★★☆☆
DIGESTION	★☆☆☆☆
SKIN	★★★☆☆

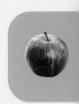

025 | grape ape

3 apples
1 bunch red grapes
1 nectarine

Very cleansing and refreshing, choose a variety of apple that contrasts with the level of sweetness of the grapes, and use a nectarine (or peach) that is ripe enough to yield to a gentle press of your thumb.

NUTRIENTS

Beta-carotene, folic acid, vitamin C, vitamin E; calcium, magnesium, manganese, phosphorus, potassium, sulphur

ENERGY	★★★★★
DETOX	★★★☆☆
IMMUNITY	★★★☆☆
DIGESTION	★☆☆☆☆
SKIN	★★★★☆

026 | parsnapple

3 apples
2 parsnips
sprinkling of grated nutmeg

I certainly turned my nose up when I first heard of the concept of juicing a parsnip, but actually, it's deliciously sweet. Blend it with a sharp apple variety. You can leave out the nutmeg if you don't feel like shaking it all up, otherwise it'll just sit on top.

NUTRIENTS

Beta-carotene, folic acid, vitamin C; calcium, magnesium, phosphorus, potassium, sodium, sulphur

ENERGY	★★★☆☆
DETOX	★★★☆☆
IMMUNITY	★★☆☆☆
DIGESTION	★☆☆☆☆
SKIN	★★★☆☆

027 | apple zing

3 apples
2 carrots
$\frac{1}{2}$ inch (1 cm) ginger root

Basic with a bite – the ginger gives a sharp snap to an otherwise sweet juice. Just snap or slice off a piece of ginger root and juice it with the other ingredients

NUTRIENTS

Beta-carotene, folic acid, vitamin C; calcium, magnesium, phosphorus, potassium, sulphur

ENERGY	★★★★☆
DETOX	★★★☆☆
IMMUNITY	★★★☆☆
DIGESTION	★★★★☆
SKIN	★★★★☆

028 | cranapple

3 apples
1 handful cranberries
1 handful grapes

Although cranberries are best known for combating urinary tract infections, they are also delicious, tangy and great for the immune system in general. Use sweet varieties of apples and grapes to offset the sharpness of the cranberries.

NUTRIENTS

Beta-carotene, folic acid, vitamin C, vitamin E; calcium, iron, magnesium, manganese, phosphorus, potassium, sulphur

ENERGY	★★★★★
DETOX	★★☆☆☆
IMMUNITY	★★★★☆
DIGESTION	★★☆☆☆
SKIN	★★★★☆

029 | prime cooler

3 apples
½ long cucumber
1 inch (2.5 cm) ginger root
1 small bunch fresh mint

There are few juice blends which are quite so refreshing — the sweetness of the apple is offset by the watery cucumber and sharpened by the ginger and mint.

NUTRIENTS

Beta-carotene, folic acid, vitamin C; calcium, magnesium, phosphorus, potassium, sodium, sulphur

ENERGY	★★☆☆☆
DETOX	★★★☆☆
IMMUNITY	★★☆☆☆
DIGESTION	★★★☆☆
SKIN	★★★☆☆

030 | bellyful

3 apples
¼ white cabbage
¼ small fennel bulb
1 small bunch fresh mint

This combination is an excellent one for soothing the digestive system. The cabbage is especially good for the stomach.

NUTRIENTS

Beta-carotene, folic acid, vitamin C, vitamin E; calcium, magnesium, phosphorus, potassium, sodium, sulphur

ENERGY	★★☆☆☆
DETOX	★★★☆☆
IMMUNITY	★★☆☆☆
DIGESTION	★★★★★
SKIN	★★★☆☆

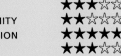

031 | pure grapefruit

3 grapefruits

Another firm favourite all on its own, whether you prefer it made with sharper white fruit or the sweeter pink or ruby varieties.

NUTRIENTS

Beta-carotene, folic acid, vitamin C; calcium, magnesium, phosphorus, potassium, sulphur

ENERGY	★★★★★
DETOX	★☆☆☆☆
IMMUNITY	★★★★☆
DIGESTION	☆☆☆☆☆
SKIN	★★☆☆☆

032 | grapefruit sharp

2 grapefruits
1 lemon
1 lime

You really will want to use sweet pink grapefruits for this one, unless you enjoy that eye-watering sourness.

NUTRIENTS

Beta-carotene, folic acid, vitamin C; calcium, magnesium, phosphorus, potassium, sodium, sulphur

ENERGY	★★★★☆
DETOX	★☆☆☆☆
IMMUNITY	★★★★★
DIGESTION	★☆☆☆☆
SKIN	★★☆☆☆

033 | grapefruit sweet

2 grapefruits
2 tangerines

I prefer using white grapefruits for this one to contrast with the sweetness of tangerines or clementines.

NUTRIENTS

Beta-carotene, folic acid, vitamin C; calcium, magnesium, phosphorus, potassium, sodium, sulphur

ENERGY	★★★★☆
DETOX	★☆☆☆☆
IMMUNITY	★★★★☆
DIGESTION	★☆☆☆☆
SKIN	★★☆☆☆

034 | grapefruit basic

1 grapefruit
1 apple
2 carrots
1 stick celery

Another one of my stock blends for a good wake-up call in the morning.

NUTRIENTS

Beta-carotene, folic acid, vitamin C;
calcium, magnesium, manganese,
phosphorus, potassium, sodium,
sulphur

ENERGY	★★★★☆
DETOX	★★★☆☆
IMMUNITY	★★★★☆
DIGESTION	★☆☆☆☆
SKIN	★★★☆☆

035 | grapefruit basic with a bite

1 grapefruit
1 apple
2 carrots
1 stick celery
$\frac{1}{2}$ inch (1 cm) ginger root

This is the Basic with a sharp kick from the ginger, particularly good
if you've got a cold.

NUTRIENTS

Beta-carotene, folic acid, vitamin C;
calcium, magnesium, manganese,
phosphorus, potassium, sodium,
sulphur

ENERGY	★★★★☆
DETOX	★★★☆☆
IMMUNITY	★★★☆☆
DIGESTION	★★☆☆☆
SKIN	★★★☆☆

036 | water cooler

2 grapefruits
1 thick slice watermelon

I have a slight preference for this over Water Cooler II (see p.54) because the
contrast of flavours and textures is even better.

NUTRIENTS

Beta-carotene, folic acid, vitamin C;
calcium, iron, magnesium, phosphorus,
potassium, sodium, sulphur

ENERGY	★★★★☆
DETOX	★★☆☆☆
IMMUNITY	★★★★☆
DIGESTION	☆☆☆☆☆
SKIN	★★★☆☆

037 | grapefruit blues

2 grapefruits
1 large handful blueberries

Whether you choose a tangy white grapefruit or sweeter pink variety,
the addition of the blueberries will transform the colour and give an
extra antioxidant lift.

NUTRIENTS

Beta-carotene, biotin, folic acid,	ENERGY	★★★★☆
vitamins B1, B2, B6, C and E; calcium,	DETOX	★★☆☆☆
chromium, magnesium, phosphorus,	IMMUNITY	★★★★★
potassium, sodium, sulphur	DIGESTION	☆☆☆☆☆
	SKIN	★★★★☆

038 | pink grapefruit

2 grapefruits
1 handful raspberries
1 handful strawberries

Just the colour of this makes you want to schlurp it up, not to mention
how great it is for your body's defences.

NUTRIENTS

Beta-carotene, biotin, folic acid,	ENERGY	★★★★☆
vitamin C; calcium, magnesium,	DETOX	★☆☆☆☆
manganese, phosphorus, potassium,	IMMUNITY	★★★★★
sodium, sulphur	DIGESTION	☆☆☆☆☆
	SKIN	★★★★☆

039 | greatfruit c

2 grapefruits
1 guava
1 kiwi

Not just for colds, high doses of vitamin C such as are found in this tasty
drink can ward off all sorts of other illnesses and aging.

NUTRIENTS

Beta-carotene, folic acid, vitamin C;	ENERGY	★★★★☆
calcium, magnesium, phosphorus,	DETOX	★★★☆☆
potassium, sodium, sulphur	IMMUNITY	★★★★★
	DIGESTION	☆☆☆☆☆
	SKIN	★★★★☆

040 | surprising sweetie

2 grapefruits
1 thick slice of melon
1 peach

You would never imagine that anything with grapefruit could be so sweet, let alone pack such an immune-boosting punch.

NUTRIENTS

Beta-carotene, folic acid, vitamin B3, vitamin C; calcium, magnesium, phosphorus, potassium, sodium, sulphur

ENERGY	★★★★☆
DETOX	★★☆☆☆
IMMUNITY	★★★★☆
DIGESTION	★★☆☆☆
SKIN	★★★★★

041 | pale faced

2 grapefruits
1 apple
½ bulb fennel
1 small bunch fresh mint

A blend of three distinctly strong flavours makes a delicious whole, with the more subtle undertones of the apple.

NUTRIENTS

Beta-carotene, folic acid, vitamin C; calcium, magnesium, phosphorus, potassium, sodium, sulphur

ENERGY	★★★★☆
DETOX	★☆☆☆☆
IMMUNITY	★★☆☆☆
DIGESTION	★★★☆☆
SKIN	★★☆☆☆

042 | grapefruit tonic

3 grapefruits
1 teaspoon spirulina

Simple but strong, the earthy taste of spirulina goes well with grapefruit. Best shaken in a jar with the juice to avoid lumps of spirulina powder.

NUTRIENTS

Beta-carotene, folic acid, vitamins B1, B3, B5, B6 and C; calcium, iron, magnesium, phosphorus, potassium, sodium, sulphur; protein; essential fatty acids

ENERGY	★★★★☆
DETOX	★★★★☆
IMMUNITY	★★★☆☆
DIGESTION	★☆☆☆☆
SKIN	★★★★☆

043 | peppery grapefruit

2 grapefruits
$\frac{1}{4}$ red cabbage

It's the strong red cabbage here which gives this juice its distinctive, peppery taste and vibrant colour.

NUTRIENTS

Beta-carotene, folic acid, vitamin C, vitamin E; calcium, magnesium, phosphorus, potassium, sodium, sulphur

ENERGY	★★★☆☆
DETOX	★☆☆☆☆
IMMUNITY	★★★★☆
DIGESTION	★★★☆☆
SKIN	★★☆☆☆

044 | orange morning

2 grapefruits
3 carrots
$\frac{1}{2}$ inch (1 cm) ginger root

Another great morning staple but one where the sharp, awakening grapefruit tang is tempered by the sweet, rich carrot.

NUTRIENTS

Beta-carotene, folic acid, vitamin C; calcium, magnesium, phosphorus, potassium, sodium, sulphur

ENERGY	★★★★☆
DETOX	★★★☆☆
IMMUNITY	★★★★☆
DIGESTION	★★★☆☆
SKIN	★★★☆☆

045 | grapefruit greens

2 grapefruits
1 handful watercress
1 bunch parsley

You can certainly taste the cleansing goodness in this one, and the strong flavour of the grapefruit can carry the greens' taste very well.

NUTRIENTS

Beta-carotene, folic acid, vitamins B3, C and E; calcium, iron, magnesium, phosphorus, potassium, sodium, sulphur

ENERGY	★★★☆☆
DETOX	★★★☆☆
IMMUNITY	★★☆☆☆
DIGESTION	★☆☆☆☆
SKIN	★★★☆☆

046 | black grapefruit

2 grapefruits
1 handful blackberries
1 handful blackcurrants

A fabulous contrast of the colours as they blend in the jug… and then a
fantastic boost to immunity. Best made in summer with fresh berries.

NUTRIENTS

Beta-carotene, folic acid, vitamins B5,
C and E; calcium, iron, magnesium,
manganese, phosphorus, potassium,
sodium, sulphur

ENERGY	★★★★☆
DETOX	★☆☆☆☆
IMMUNITY	★★★★★
DIGESTION	☆☆☆☆☆
SKIN	★★★★☆

047 | cloudy day

2 grapefruits
½ long cucumber
2 sticks celery
1 small bunch fresh mint

The sweet tang of the grapefruit contrasts wonderfully with the almost
melon-like cucumber and salty celery, all lifted by the mint.

NUTRIENTS

Beta-carotene, folic acid, vitamin C;
calcium, magnesium, phosphorus,
potassium, sodium, sulphur

ENERGY	★★★☆☆
DETOX	★★☆☆☆
IMMUNITY	★★☆☆☆
DIGESTION	★★☆☆☆
SKIN	★★☆☆☆

048 | bleeding grapefruit

2 grapefruits
2 sticks celery
½ beet (beetroot)

The earthy sweetness of the beet nicely balances the sharpness of white grapefruit, while the salty celery brings out all the flavours.

NUTRIENTS

Beta-carotene, folic acid, vitamin C; calcium, magnesium, manganese, phosphorus, potassium, sodium, sulphur

ENERGY	★★★☆☆
DETOX	★★★★☆
IMMUNITY	★★☆☆☆
DIGESTION	★☆☆☆☆
SKIN	★★★☆☆

049 | tangy veggie

2 grapefruits
2 inches (5 cm) sweet potato
1 parsnip
1 stick celery

Another great combination of sweet, earthy root vegetables and sharp, white grapefruit, or pink if you prefer. The celery serves to magnify the flavours further.

NUTRIENTS

Beta-carotene, folic acid, vitamin C, vitamin E; calcium, magnesium, manganese, phosphorus, potassium, sodium, sulphur

ENERGY	★★★☆☆
DETOX	★★★☆☆
IMMUNITY	★★☆☆☆
DIGESTION	★☆☆☆☆
SKIN	★★☆☆☆

050 | grapefruit cold zap

2 grapefruits
1 lemon
1 inch (2.5 cm) ginger root
1 clove garlic

You'd only really want this one if you were full of cold, unless you're trying to keep vampires away.

NUTRIENTS

Beta-carotene, folic acid, vitamin C; calcium, magnesium, phosphorus, potassium, sulphur

ENERGY	★★★☆☆
DETOX	★★☆☆☆
IMMUNITY	★★★★★
DIGESTION	★★☆☆☆
SKIN	★★★☆☆

051 | the original juice

4 oranges

Pure OJ is certainly the number one juice in the West, but not even
the so-called "freshly squeezed" juices come close to making your own
and drinking it immediately.

NUTRIENTS

Beta-carotene, vitamin C; calcium,
magnesium, phosphorus, potassium

ENERGY	★★★★☆
DETOX	★☆☆☆☆
IMMUNITY	★★★★☆
DIGESTION	☆☆☆☆☆
SKIN	★★☆☆☆

052 | bloodthirst

6 blood oranges

A winter speciality, sweet, red blood oranges remind me of rare trips
to my family home in Malta in the winter. You can often find them in
supermarkets – particularly small, juicy organic ones. Best left
unadulterated by other fruits.

NUTRIENTS

Beta-carotene, vitamin C; calcium,
magnesium, phosphorus, potassium

ENERGY	★★★★☆
DETOX	★☆☆☆☆
IMMUNITY	★★★★☆
DIGESTION	☆☆☆☆☆
SKIN	★★☆☆☆

053 | orange basic

2 oranges
1 apple
3 carrots
1 stick celery
1 inch (2 cm) ginger root

One of my everyday staples – it doesn't require too much imagination
as most refrigerators and fruit bowls will have the ingredients.

NUTRIENTS

Beta-carotene, folic acid, vitamin C;
calcium, magnesium, manganese,
phosphorus, potassium, sodium,
sulphur

ENERGY	★★★★☆
DETOX	★★★★☆
IMMUNITY	★★★★☆
DIGESTION	★★☆☆☆
SKIN	★★★☆☆

054 | bright orange

2 oranges
4 carrots

Even easier than the Basic, the incredible colour of this simple combination heralds an equally amazing taste.

NUTRIENTS

Beta-carotene, folic acid, vitamin C; calcium, magnesium, phosphorus, potassium, sodium, sulphur

ENERGY	★★★★☆
DETOX	★★★☆☆
IMMUNITY	★★★★☆
DIGESTION	★☆☆☆☆
SKIN	★★★☆☆

055 | florida blue

2 oranges
1 pink grapefruit
1 handful blueberries

If you use a sweet pink grapefruit, rather than a sharper white one, this blend is divine.

NUTRIENTS

Beta-carotene, biotin, folic acid, vitamins B1, B2, B6, C and E; calcium, magnesium, phosphorus, potassium, sodium, sulphur

ENERGY	★★★★☆
DETOX	★☆☆☆☆
IMMUNITY	★★★★★
DIGESTION	★★☆☆☆
SKIN	★★★☆☆

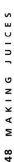

056 | orange crudités

2 oranges
½ long cucumber
2 carrots
1 stick celery

The three vegetables in this juice gently dilute the sweet, sharp
taste of oranges, and make it a lighter, more refreshing drink.

NUTRIENTS

Beta-carotene, folic acid, vitamin C;
calcium, magnesium, manganese,
phosphorus, potassium, sodium, sulphur

ENERGY	★★★☆☆
DETOX	★★☆☆☆
IMMUNITY	★★★☆☆
DIGESTION	★★☆☆☆
SKIN	★★★☆☆

057 | power packed c

3 oranges
1 guava
1 handful strawberries

With three of the richest sources of vitamin C mixed together,
this is not only a delicious drink but is also a strong immune
booster that helps keep illnesses at bay.

NUTRIENTS

Beta-carotene, biotin, folic acid,
vitamin B3, vitamin C; calcium,
magnesium, phosphorus, potassium,
sodium, sulphur

ENERGY	★★★★★
DETOX	★☆☆☆☆
IMMUNITY	★★★★★
DIGESTION	☆☆☆☆☆
SKIN	★★★★☆

058 | william's orange

2 oranges
2 pears

You'd think the pears would get swamped by the oranges in this juice, but, in fact, they just tone down the tang beautifully. It's best to use a sweet variety of pear such as Williams.

NUTRIENTS

Beta-carotene, folic acid, vitamin C;
calcium, magnesium, phosphorus,
potassium, sulphur

ENERGY	★★★★☆
DETOX	★☆☆☆☆
IMMUNITY	★★★☆☆
DIGESTION	★☆☆☆☆
SKIN	★☆☆☆☆

059 | orange medley

2 oranges
½ melon
1 nectarine

Use a cantaloupe melon to make this a wonderful blend of orange-coloured fruits.

NUTRIENTS

Beta-carotene, folic acid, vitamin C;
calcium, magnesium, phosphorus,
potassium, sodium

ENERGY	★★★★★
DETOX	★☆☆☆☆
IMMUNITY	★★★★★
DIGESTION	★★☆☆☆
SKIN	★★★★☆

060 | citrus sweet

2 oranges
3 tangerines

This juice really highlights the differences between the tastes of oranges and the smaller tangerine or other similar fruits. Clementines or any small, easily peeled orange citrus fruits may be used.

NUTRIENTS

Beta-carotene, folic acid, vitamin C;
calcium, magnesium, phosphorus,
potassium, sodium

ENERGY	★★★★☆
DETOX	★☆☆☆☆
IMMUNITY	★★★★☆
DIGESTION	☆☆☆☆☆
SKIN	☆☆☆☆☆

061 | biting orange

4 oranges
½ inch (1 cm) ginger root

Almost any juice goes well with ginger in my book, but this sweet orange with a ginger bite giving it a festive winter flavour is a particular favourite.

NUTRIENTS

Beta-carotene, vitamin C, calcium; magnesium, phosphorus, potassium

ENERGY	★★★★☆
DETOX	☆☆☆☆☆
IMMUNITY	★★★★☆
DIGESTION	★★☆☆☆
SKIN	★☆☆☆☆

062 | bitter melon

2 oranges
2 thick slices of melon

Bitter Melon is actually the name of an Indian vegetable (and a 90s American rock band), but also sums up this juice's tangy twist on sweet melon. Use a cantaloupe or honeydew melon.

NUTRIENTS

Beta-carotene, folic acid, vitamin C; calcium, magnesium, phosphorus, potassium, sodium, sulphur

ENERGY	★★★★★
DETOX	★☆☆☆☆
IMMUNITY	★★★★★
DIGESTION	☆☆☆☆☆
SKIN	★★★★☆

063 | orange winter crumble

2 oranges
2 apples
1 handful blackberries

I love the blend of orange juice with the traditional winter mixture of apple and blackberry used in pies and crumbles.

NUTRIENTS

Beta-carotene, folic acid, vitamin C, vitamin E; calcium, iron, magnesium, manganese, phosphorus, potassium, sodium, sulphur

ENERGY	★★★★★
DETOX	★★☆☆☆
IMMUNITY	★★★★★
DIGESTION	★☆☆☆☆
SKIN	★★★★☆

064 | citrus sharp

3 oranges
1 lemon
1 lime

The colour of this refreshing juice hails a tart
tickling of the tastebuds, and all that citrus fruit
gives you a great immune boost.

NUTRIENTS

Beta-carotene, folic acid, vitamin C;
calcium, magnesium, phosphorus,
potassium, sodium, sulphur

ENERGY	★★★★☆
DETOX	★☆☆☆☆
IMMUNITY	★★★★★
DIGESTION	☆☆☆☆☆
SKIN	★★☆☆☆

065 | muddy puddle

3 oranges
1 handful spinach
1 handful watercress
2 broccoli florets

The name of this originates from a drink a friend of mind used to have
at college – orange juice and cola. But it's a far cry from that in terms of
sweetness and health properties. The strength of flavour of the oranges
carries the earthy, strong taste of the greens.

NUTRIENTS

Beta-carotene, vitamin B5, vitamin C;
calcium, magnesium, phosphorus,
potassium, sodium

ENERGY	★★★☆☆
DETOX	★★★★☆
IMMUNITY	★★★☆☆
DIGESTION	★☆☆☆☆
SKIN	★★★☆☆

066 | blackcurrant twist

3 oranges
1 handful blackcurrants
$\frac{1}{4}$ fennel bulb

This always reminds me of a tangy version of blackcurrant and aniseed sweets I would buy as a child.

NUTRIENTS

Beta-carotene, biotin, vitamins B5,	ENERGY	★★★☆☆
C and E; calcium, magnesium,	DETOX	☆☆☆☆☆
phosphorus, potassium, sodium,	IMMUNITY	★★★☆☆
sulphur	DIGESTION	☆☆☆☆☆
	SKIN	★★☆☆☆

067 | muddy tonic

4 oranges
1 teaspoon spirulina

I love the earthy green taste mixed with orange, although the brown colour isn't the most appealing. It's best to shake the juice (or a portion of it) with the spirulina in a jar so it doesn't go lumpy.

NUTRIENTS

Beta-carotene, vitamins B1, B3, B5,	ENERGY	★★★☆☆
B6 and C; calcium, iron, magnesium,	DETOX	★★★☆☆
phosphorus, potassium, sodium;	IMMUNITY	★★☆☆☆
protein, essential fatty acids	DIGESTION	☆☆☆☆☆
	SKIN	★★☆☆☆

068 | bloody orange

3 oranges
1 beet (beetroot)

The name is a reference to this juice's thick red colour and not to blood oranges which are, unfortunately, all too rare – the earthy taste of beet cuts through the sharpness of good oranges well.

NUTRIENTS

Beta-carotene, folic acid, vitamin C;	ENERGY	★★★☆☆
calcium, magnesium, phosphorus,	DETOX	★★☆☆☆
potassium, sodium	IMMUNITY	★★★☆☆
	DIGESTION	☆☆☆☆☆
	SKIN	★★★☆☆

069 | orange aniseed twist

3 oranges
2 sticks celery
¼ fennel bulb

The fennel gives a great turn to this recipe, while the saltiness of the celery brings out the flavours. All in all, very refreshing.

NUTRIENTS

Beta-carotene, folic acid, vitamin C; calcium, magnesium, manganese, phosphorus, potassium, sodium, sulphur

ENERGY	★★★☆☆
DETOX	★☆☆☆☆
IMMUNITY	★☆☆☆☆
DIGESTION	★★★☆☆
SKIN	★☆☆☆☆

070 | water cooler II

3 oranges
1 thick slice watermelon

Unbelievably light and refreshing, the watermelon takes the edge off the tangy orange.

NUTRIENTS

Beta-carotene, vitamin C; calcium, iron, magnesium, phosphorus, potassium, sodium, sulphur

ENERGY	★★★★☆
DETOX	★★☆☆☆
IMMUNITY	★★★☆☆
DIGESTION	☆☆☆☆☆
SKIN	★★★★☆

071 | orange pepper

3 oranges
½ red or yellow bell pepper
1 kale leaf
1 handful watercress

The strong taste of oranges carries the more subtle tastes of the vegetables in this juice. Don't be put off by the muddy colour.

NUTRIENTS

Beta-carotene, folic acid, vitamins B3, C and E; calcium, iron, magnesium, manganese, phosphorus, potassium, sodium, sulphur

ENERGY	★★☆☆☆
DETOX	★★★☆☆
IMMUNITY	★★★☆☆
DIGESTION	★★☆☆☆
SKIN	★★★★☆

072 | orange blush

3 oranges
1 apple
1 handful raspberries

A tangy pink juice which blends three fantastic fruits perfectly — definitely greater than the sum of its parts.

NUTRIENTS

Beta-carotene, biotin, folic acid, vitamin C; calcium, magnesium, manganese, phosphorus, potassium, sodium, sulphur

ENERGY	★★★★★
DETOX	★☆☆☆☆
IMMUNITY	★★★☆☆
DIGESTION	★☆☆☆☆
SKIN	★★★☆☆

073 | counteractor

3 oranges
$\frac{1}{4}$ red cabbage
$\frac{1}{4}$ inch (0.5 cm) ginger root

Some people find oranges too acidic on their digestion — here the soothing cabbage and ginger provide the perfect balance.

NUTRIENTS

Beta-carotene, folic acid, vitamin C, vitamin E; calcium, magnesium, phosphorus, potassium, sodium

ENERGY	★★★☆☆
DETOX	★☆☆☆☆
IMMUNITY	★★☆☆☆
DIGESTION	★★★☆☆
SKIN	★★☆☆☆

074 | pure raspberry

2 large handfuls raspberries

For the vast majority of us an absurd luxury, so make just a small
glassful and savour every drop.

NUTRIENTS

Beta-carotene, biotin, vitamin C; calcium,
magnesium, manganese, phosphorus,
potassium, sodium, sulphur

ENERGY	★★★★★
DETOX	★☆☆☆☆
IMMUNITY	★★★☆☆
DIGESTION	☆☆☆☆☆
SKIN	★★★☆☆

075 | raspapple

2 large handfuls raspberries
2 large apples

A simple but splendid blend of juices.

NUTRIENTS

Beta-carotene, biotin, folic acid,
vitamin C; calcium, magnesium,
manganese, phosphorus, potassium,
sodium, sulphur

ENERGY	★★★★★
DETOX	★☆☆☆☆
IMMUNITY	★★☆☆☆
DIGESTION	★☆☆☆☆
SKIN	★★★☆☆

076 | raspapple tang

2 large handfuls raspberries
2 large apples
1 lime

Remarkably different with just the addition of a little lime.

NUTRIENTS

Beta-carotene, biotin, folic acid,
vitamin C; calcium, magnesium,
manganese, phosphorus, potassium,
sodium, sulphur

ENERGY	★★★★☆
DETOX	★☆☆☆☆
IMMUNITY	★★★★☆
DIGESTION	★☆☆☆☆
SKIN	★★☆☆☆

077 | citrusberry

2 large handfuls raspberries
2 large oranges
1 tangerine

This is such a classic, delicious blend, they even sell it in supermarkets without the tangerine, which I find just tones it down a nice touch.

NUTRIENTS

Beta-carotene, biotin, vitamin C; calcium, magnesium, manganese, phosphorus, potassium, sodium, sulphur

ENERGY	★★★★★
DETOX	★☆☆☆☆
IMMUNITY	★★★★☆
DIGESTION	☆☆☆☆☆
SKIN	★★★☆☆

078 | sharp citrusberry

2 large handfuls raspberries
1 grapefruit
½ lemon

I almost prefer this one to the orange blend (see above), with the bite of the grapefruit and the nose-curling lemon.

NUTRIENTS

Beta-carotene, folic acid, biotin, vitamin C; calcium, magnesium, manganese, phosphorus, potassium, sodium, sulphur

ENERGY	★★★★☆
DETOX	★☆☆☆☆
IMMUNITY	★★★☆☆
DIGESTION	☆☆☆☆☆
SKIN	★★★☆☆

079 | creamy raspberry

2 large handfuls raspberries
½ melon
1 stick celery

With the creaminess of the melon, you'd think you were drinking more than just fruit juice, while the salty celery lifts all the flavours.

NUTRIENTS

Beta-carotene, biotin, folic acid, vitamin C; calcium, magnesium, manganese, phosphorus, potassium, sodium, sulphur

ENERGY	★★★★★
DETOX	★☆☆☆☆
IMMUNITY	★★★☆☆
DIGESTION	☆☆☆☆☆
SKIN	★★★★☆

080 | gently raspberry

2 large handfuls raspberries
2 pears
$\frac{1}{4}$ cucumber

Not quite as strange a combination as you may initially think – the cucumber in this appears to save the pears from being drowned out by the raspberries.

NUTRIENTS

Beta-carotene, biotin, folic acid, vitamin C; calcium, magnesium, manganese, phosphorus, potassium, sodium, sulphur

ENERGY	★★★☆☆
DETOX	★☆☆☆☆
IMMUNITY	★★☆☆☆
DIGESTION	★☆☆☆☆
SKIN	★★☆☆☆

081 | raspberry sensation

2 large handfuls raspberries
$\frac{1}{2}$ pineapple

A truly sensational combination — go on, spoil yourself with two independently rich fruits laden with goodness.

NUTRIENTS

Beta-carotene, biotin, folic acid, vitamin C; calcium, magnesium, manganese phosphorus, potassium, sodium, sulphur

ENERGY	★★★★★
DETOX	★☆☆☆☆
IMMUNITY	★★☆☆☆
DIGESTION	★★★★☆
SKIN	★★★☆☆

082 | berry bonanza

2 large handfuls raspberries
1 handful blackcurrants
1 handful blueberries

Taking the luxury even
further …this berry combination
is a blessing to your tastebuds
and your body.

NUTRIENTS

Beta-carotene, biotin, folic acid,
vitamins B1, B2, B5, B6, C and E;
calcium, chromium, magnesium,
phosphorus, potassium, sodium,
sulphur

ENERGY	★★★★★
DETOX	★☆☆☆☆
IMMUNITY	★★★★★
DIGESTION	☆☆☆☆☆
SKIN	★★★★☆

083 | morning berry basic

2 large handfuls raspberries
2 apples
1 orange
1 teaspoon spirulina

Fruit bowl classics with the raspberries and some spirulina for an
extra health kick. To avoid green lumps, shake the spirulina in a jar
with a little of the juice before mixing it in with the rest.

NUTRIENTS

Beta-carotene, vitamins B1, B3, B5, B6 and C;
calcium, iron, magnesium, manganese,
phosphorus, potassium, sodium, sulphur;
protein, essential fatty acids

ENERGY	★★★★☆
DETOX	★★★★☆
IMMUNITY	★★★☆☆
DIGESTION	★☆☆☆☆
SKIN	★★★★☆

084 | pure peach

4 peaches or nectarines

Pure heaven for anyone with the slightest penchant for fruit of any sort.

NUTRIENTS

Beta-carotene, folic acid, vitamin B3, vitamin C; calcium, magnesium, phosphorus, potassium, sodium, sulphur

ENERGY	★★★★★
DETOX	★☆☆☆☆
IMMUNITY	★★★★☆
DIGESTION	★★☆☆☆
SKIN	★★★★☆

085 | eve's peach

2 peaches or nectarines
2 apples

I'm sure the serpent would not have had to do much persuading for this one!

NUTRIENTS

Beta-carotene, folic acid, vitamin B3, vitamin C; calcium, magnesium, phosphorus, potassium, sodium, sulphur

ENERGY	★★★★★
DETOX	★☆☆☆☆
IMMUNITY	★★★★☆
DIGESTION	★★☆☆☆
SKIN	★★★★☆

086 | peach 'n' pine

2 peaches or nectarines
½ pineapple

Tropical and temperate, tangy and delicate.

NUTRIENTS

Beta-carotene, folic acid, vitamin B3, vitamin C; calcium, magnesium, manganese, phosphorus, potassium, sodium, sulphur

ENERGY	★★★★★
DETOX	★☆☆☆☆
IMMUNITY	★★★☆☆
DIGESTION	★★★☆☆
SKIN	★★★☆☆

087 | black peach

2 peaches or nectarines
2 handfuls blueberries, blackberries and/or blackcurrants

A summer delight – each drop to be savoured. Play with the different berry combinations to change the flavour and the sweetness.

NUTRIENTS

Beta-carotene, biotin, folic acid, vitamins B1, B2, B3, B6, C and E; calcium, chromium, iron, magnesium, manganese, phosphorus, potassium, sodium, sulphur

ENERGY	★★★★★
DETOX	★★☆☆☆
IMMUNITY	★★★★☆
DIGESTION	★☆☆☆☆
SKIN	★★★★★

088 | pink peach

2 peaches or nectarines
2 handfuls strawberries and raspberries

Another exquisite summer luxury – choose your favourite combination.

NUTRIENTS

Beta-carotene, biotin, folic acid, vitamin B3, vitamin C; calcium, magnesium, phosphorus, potassium, sodium, sulphur

ENERGY	★★★★★
DETOX	★★☆☆☆
IMMUNITY	★★★★☆
DIGESTION	★☆☆☆☆
SKIN	★★★★★

089 | peaches and cream

2 peaches or nectarines
$\frac{1}{2}$ melon

If any creamless drink comes close to peaches and cream this delicious concoction is it.

NUTRIENTS

Beta-carotene, folic acid, vitamin B3, vitamin C; calcium, magnesium, phosphorus, potassium, sodium, sulphur

ENERGY	★★★★★
DETOX	★☆☆☆☆
IMMUNITY	★★★★☆
DIGESTION	★☆☆☆☆
SKIN	★★★★☆

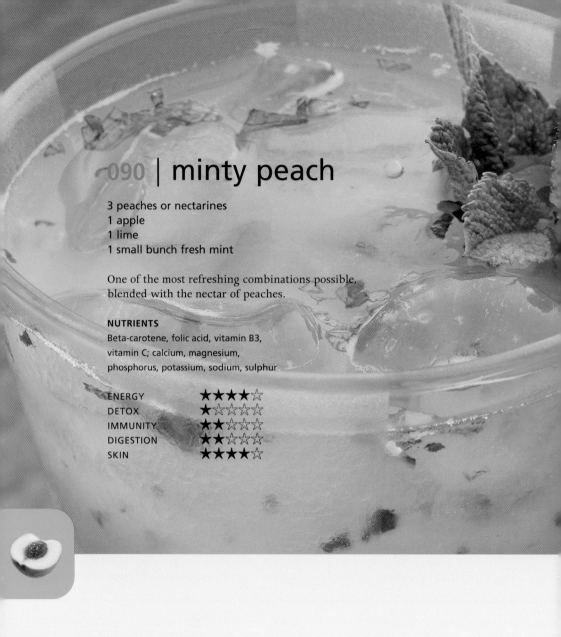

090 | minty peach

3 peaches or nectarines
1 apple
1 lime
1 small bunch fresh mint

One of the most refreshing combinations possible,
blended with the nectar of peaches.

NUTRIENTS

Beta-carotene, folic acid, vitamin B3,
vitamin C; calcium, magnesium,
phosphorus, potassium, sodium, sulphur

ENERGY	★★★★☆
DETOX	★☆☆☆☆
IMMUNITY	★★☆☆☆
DIGESTION	★★☆☆☆
SKIN	★★★★☆

091 | peaches and green

3 peaches or nectarines
2 sticks celery
1 teaspoon spirulina

Even the less inviting earthiness of the celery and spirulina are forgotten
in this super-healthy blend. To avoid green lumps, shake the spirulina in
a jar with a little of the juice before mixing it in with the rest.

NUTRIENTS

Beta-carotene, folic acid, vitamin B3,
vitamin C; calcium, magnesium, manganese,
phosphorus, potassium, sodium, sulphur;
protein, essential fatty acids

ENERGY	★★★☆☆
DETOX	★★★★☆
IMMUNITY	★★☆☆☆
DIGESTION	★☆☆☆☆
SKIN	★★★★☆

092 | tangerine cream

3 peaches or nectarines
2 tangerines or clementines

When oranges simply won't do – only the delicate taste of tangerine or any similar citrus fruit. Combine with peach or nectarine and you get a creamy, sweet blend.

NUTRIENTS

Beta-carotene, folic acid, vitamin B3, vitamin C; calcium, magnesium, phosphorus, potassium, sodium, sulphur

ENERGY	★★★★★
DETOX	★☆☆☆☆
IMMUNITY	★★★★★
DIGESTION	★☆☆☆☆
SKIN	★★★★☆

093 | sunset peach

2 peaches or nectarines
1 apple
2 carrots
1 handful raspberries

The carrots add a surprising creamy sweetness to this one and can even make up for getting a dud batch of raspberries that aren't that sweet.

NUTRIENTS

Beta-carotene, biotin, folic acid, vitamin B3, vitamin C; calcium, magnesium, manganese, phosphorus, potassium, sodium, sulphur

ENERGY	★★★★★
DETOX	★★☆☆☆
IMMUNITY	★★★★★
DIGESTION	★★☆☆☆
SKIN	★★★★☆

094 | cherry pie

2 large handfuls cherries
2 apples

Nothing to do with pies at all, but the sweetness of apples blends beautifully with the cherries.

NUTRIENTS

Beta-carotene, folic acid, vitamin C;
calcium, magnesium, phosphorus,
potassium, sodium, sulphur

ENERGY	★★★★★
DETOX	★★★☆☆
IMMUNITY	★★★★☆
DIGESTION	★★☆☆☆
SKIN	★★★☆☆

095 | citrus cherry

2 large handfuls cherries
2 oranges
$\frac{1}{2}$ lime

You'll be hard pressed to enjoy a better combination with orange juice as this one.

NUTRIENTS

Beta-carotene, folic acid, vitamin C;
calcium, magnesium, phosphorus,
potassium, sodium, sulphur

ENERGY	★★★★★
DETOX	★☆☆☆☆
IMMUNITY	★★★★☆
DIGESTION	★☆☆☆☆
SKIN	★★★★☆

096 | sweet cherry pine

2 large handfuls cherries
$\frac{1}{2}$ pineapple

The combination of these two fruits produces an unbelievable sensation of intense taste and texture with the rich sweetness of the cherries and the pineapple's tang.

NUTRIENTS

Beta-carotene, folic acid, vitamin C;
calcium, magnesium, manganese,
phosphorus, potassium, sodium, sulphur

ENERGY	★★★★☆
DETOX	★★☆☆☆
IMMUNITY	★★★★☆
DIGESTION	★★★☆☆
SKIN	★★★★☆

097 | thicker than water

2 large handfuls cherries
2 apples
$\frac{1}{2}$ beet (beetroot)

The colour of this smooth, sumptuous juice almost makes you
want to hold it as though it were a soft, pink velvet.

NUTRIENTS
Beta-carotene, folic acid,
vitamin C; calcium,
magnesium, phosphorus,
potassium, sodium, sulphur

ENERGY	★★★★★
DETOX	★★★☆☆
IMMUNITY	★★★★☆
DIGESTION	★★★☆☆
SKIN	★★★★☆

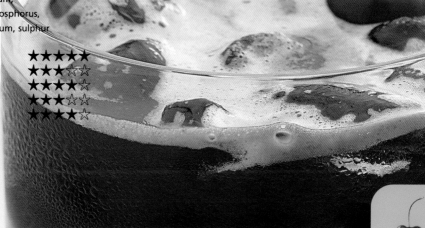

098 | cherry cooler

2 large handfuls cherries
$\frac{1}{2}$ long cucumber
2 sticks celery

This may seem like a peculiar combination but the cucumber and celery
provide delicious light relief from the density of the cherry juice.

NUTRIENTS
Beta-carotene, folic acid, vitamin C;
calcium, magnesium, manganese,
phosphorus, potassium, sodium, sulphur

ENERGY	★★★☆☆
DETOX	★★☆☆☆
IMMUNITY	★★★☆☆
DIGESTION	★★☆☆☆
SKIN	★★☆☆☆

099 | pure pear

4 pears

In addition to some of the tropical fruits, I think a ripe Williams pear ranks right up there as one of my favourites.

NUTRIENTS

Beta-carotene, folic acid, vitamin C; calcium, magnesium, phosphorus, potassium, sulphur

ENERGY	★★★★☆
DETOX	★★☆☆☆
IMMUNITY	★☆☆☆☆
DIGESTION	★★★☆☆
SKIN	★★☆☆☆

100 | pear basic

2 pears
1 apple
2 carrots
½ inch (1 cm) ginger root

A good, standard morning blend to set you up for the day ahead.

NUTRIENTS

Beta-carotene, folic acid, vitamin C; calcium, magnesium, phosphorus, potassium, sodium, sulphur

ENERGY	★★★★☆
DETOX	★★★☆☆
IMMUNITY	★★★☆☆
DIGESTION	★★☆☆☆
SKIN	★★★☆☆

101 | pear tart

4 pears
½ inch (1 cm) ginger root
¼ teaspoon cinnamon powder

Pears go so well with a gentle hint of spices. The cinnamon is best shaken up with the juice in a jar after it's made.

NUTRIENTS

Beta-carotene, folic acid, vitamin C; calcium, magnesium, phosphorus, potassium, sulphur

ENERGY	★★★★☆
DETOX	★☆☆☆☆
IMMUNITY	★★★☆☆
DIGESTION	★★★☆☆
SKIN	★☆☆☆☆

102 | blue pear

2 pears
1 handful blueberries
1 handful blackberries

The sweetness of all three of these fruits is divine.

NUTRIENTS

Beta-carotene, biotin, folic acid,	ENERGY	★★★★☆
vitamins B1, B2, B6, C, E; calcium,	DETOX	★★★☆☆
chromium, iron, magnesium,	IMMUNITY	★★★★☆
manganese, phosphorus, potassium,	DIGESTION	★☆☆☆☆
sodium, sulphur	SKIN	★★★☆☆

103 | black pear

3 pears
1 handful blackcurrants

Quite distinct from Blue Pear, the sweet sharpness of the blackcurrants blends wonderfully with pears.

NUTRIENTS

Beta-carotene, folic acid, biotin,	ENERGY	★★★★☆
vitamins B5, C and E; calcium,	DETOX	★★★☆☆
magnesium, phosphorus, potassium,	IMMUNITY	★★★★☆
sodium, sulphur	DIGESTION	★☆☆☆☆
	SKIN	★★★☆☆

104 | pink pear

2 pears
1 handful raspberries
1 handful strawberries

In my view, raspberries and strawberries go well with pretty much any fruit, and this is certainly no exception.

NUTRIENTS

Beta-carotene, biotin, folic acid,	ENERGY	★★★★★
vitamin C; calcium, magnesium,	DETOX	★★☆☆☆
manganese, phosphorus, potassium,	IMMUNITY	★★★★☆
sodium, sulphur	DIGESTION	★☆☆☆☆
	SKIN	★★★☆☆

105 | pink pear II

3 pears
1 handful cranberries

Another bright pink juice, this one is fantastic for the immune system, particularly for urinary-tract infections. Unless you want a very sharp taste, make sure you use nearly ripe Williams pears.

NUTRIENTS

Beta-carotene, folic acid, vitamin C; calcium, iron, magnesium, phosphorus, potassium, sodium, sulphur

ENERGY	★★★☆☆
DETOX	★★☆☆☆
IMMUNITY	★★★★☆
DIGESTION	★☆☆☆☆
SKIN	★★★☆☆

106 | tangerine dream

3 pears
2 tangerines

Although pears go well with any citrus fruit, the slightly more delicate flavour of tangerine or clementine really draws out the taste of the pear.

NUTRIENTS

Beta-carotene, folic acid, vitamin C; calcium, magnesium, phosphorus, potassium, sodium, sulphur

ENERGY	★★★★☆
DETOX	★★☆☆☆
IMMUNITY	★★★☆☆
DIGESTION	★☆☆☆☆
SKIN	★★★☆☆

107 | big c pear

2 pears
2 kiwis
2 guavas

These two vitamin C-packed fruits create a divine taste with pear.

NUTRIENTS

Beta-carotene, folic acid, vitamin B3, vitamin C; calcium, magnesium, phosphorus, potassium, sodium, sulphur

ENERGY	★★★★★
DETOX	★★☆☆☆
IMMUNITY	★★★★★
DIGESTION	★★☆☆☆
SKIN	★★★★☆

108 | creamy pear

3 pears
1 thick slice melon
1 small bunch fresh mint

The taste and texture of melon juice somehow conjures up the sensation of creaminess.

NUTRIENTS

Beta-carotene, folic acid, vitamin C;
calcium, magnesium, phosphorus,
potassium, sodium, sulphur

ENERGY	★★★★☆
DETOX	★☆☆☆☆
IMMUNITY	★★★★☆
DIGESTION	★★☆☆☆
SKIN	★★★☆☆

109 | tropical pear

3 pears
$\frac{1}{4}$ pineapple
$\frac{1}{2}$ lime

Perhaps two of my favourite fruits with a hint of tangy lime.

NUTRIENTS

Beta-carotene, folic acid, vitamin C;
calcium, magnesium, manganese,
phosphorus, potassium, sodium,
sulphur

ENERGY	★★★★☆
DETOX	★★☆☆☆
IMMUNITY	★★★★☆
DIGESTION	★★★☆☆
SKIN	★★☆☆☆

110 | pear dream

3 pears
4 apricots

Two delicate, gentle flavours bound to create a dreamy combination.

NUTRIENTS

Beta-carotene, folic acid, vitamin C;
calcium, magnesium, phosphorus,
potassium, sulphur

ENERGY	★★★★☆
DETOX	★★☆☆☆
IMMUNITY	★★★★☆
DIGESTION	★★☆☆☆
SKIN	★★★★☆

111 | breakfast pear

3 pears
2 sticks celery
$\frac{1}{2}$ inch (1 cm) ginger root

The saltiness of celery and the hot bite of the ginger make this a great morning recipe for awakening the tastebuds.

NUTRIENTS

Beta-carotene, folic acid, vitamin C; calcium, magnesium, phosphorus, potassium, sodium, sulphur

ENERGY	★★★☆☆
DETOX	★★★★☆
IMMUNITY	★★★☆☆
DIGESTION	★★☆☆☆
SKIN	★☆☆☆☆

112 | fresh pear

3 pears
$\frac{1}{2}$ long cucumber
small bunch fresh mint

There aren't many juices like that of a cucumber to quench your thirst and combined with pear and then the mint too … mmm.

NUTRIENTS

Beta-carotene, folic acid, vitamin C; calcium, magnesium, phosphorus, potassium, sodium, sulphur

ENERGY	★★★☆☆
DETOX	★★★★☆
IMMUNITY	★☆☆☆☆
DIGESTION	★★☆☆☆
SKIN	★★☆☆☆

113 | gut soother

2 pears
2 carrots
$\frac{1}{2}$ pineapple
$\frac{1}{2}$ inch (1 cm) ginger root

The blend of these three along with the ginger not only make a great taste, but they're good for the digestive tract too.

NUTRIENTS

Beta-carotene, folic acid, vitamin C; calcium, magnesium, manganese, phosphorus, potassium, sodium, sulphur

ENERGY	★★★☆☆
DETOX	★★☆☆☆
IMMUNITY	★★★☆☆
DIGESTION	★★★★★
SKIN	★★★☆☆

114 | pure pineapple

1 pineapple

It was always my favourite juice in a can, bottle or carton ... until
I discovered the real thing.

NUTRIENTS

Beta-carotene, folic acid, vitamin C;
calcium, magnesium, manganese,
phosphorus, potassium, sodium

ENERGY	★★★★★
DETOX	★★★☆☆
IMMUNITY	★★★☆☆
DIGESTION	★★★★★
SKIN	★★★☆☆

115 | pineapple tang

1 pineapple
1 lime

Mixed with lime, pineapple takes me straight to the streets of Bangkok.

NUTRIENTS

Beta-carotene, folic acid, vitamin C;
calcium, magnesium, manganese,
phosphorus, potassium, sodium,
sulphur

ENERGY	★★★★★
DETOX	★★★☆☆
IMMUNITY	★★★☆☆
DIGESTION	★★★★★
SKIN	★★★☆☆

116 | pink pineapple

$\frac{1}{2}$ pineapple
1 handful raspberries
1 handful strawberries

This rich yet fresh juice is a beautiful shade of pink created by a blend
of tropical and temperate climes.

NUTRIENTS

Beta-carotene, biotin, folic acid,
vitamin C; calcium, magnesium,
manganese, phosphorus, potassium,
sodium, sulphur

ENERGY	★★★★★
DETOX	★☆☆☆☆
IMMUNITY	★★★★☆
DIGESTION	★★★☆☆
SKIN	★★★☆☆

117 | black pineapple

½ pineapple
1 handful blackcurrants
1 handful blackberries

Another tropic-temperate blend of fruits which goes down perfectly.

NUTRIENTS

Beta-carotene, biotin, folic acid,
vitamins B5, C and E; calcium, iron,
magnesium, manganese, phosphorus,
potassium, sodium, sulphur

ENERGY	★★★★★
DETOX	★★☆☆☆
IMMUNITY	★★★★☆
DIGESTION	★★★☆☆
SKIN	★★★★☆

118 | sweet sunset

½ pineapple
1 thick slice watermelon

The watery sweetness of the melon contrasts ideally with the rich tang
of pineapple in this all-round health-affirming, thirst-quenching drink.

NUTRIENTS

Beta-carotene, folic acid, vitamin B5,
vitamin C; calcium, magnesium,
manganese, phosphorus, potassium,
sodium

ENERGY	★★★★★
DETOX	★★★★☆
IMMUNITY	★★★★☆
DIGESTION	★★☆☆☆
SKIN	★★★★☆

119 | aniseed black

½ pineapple
1 large handful blackcurrants
½ fennel bulb

A stark reminder of blackcurrant and aniseed boiled candy with
a tangy difference.

NUTRIENTS

Beta-carotene, biotin, folic acid,
vitamins B5, C and E; calcium,
magnesium, manganese, phosphorus,
potassium, sodium, sulphur

ENERGY	★★★★☆
DETOX	★☆☆☆☆
IMMUNITY	★★★☆☆
DIGESTION	★★★★☆
SKIN	★★★★☆

120 | ginger zinger

½ pineapple
2 oranges
1 inch (2.5 cm) ginger root

One of the most refreshing, tangy combinations there is. You could add more ginger if you're a real fan and get an even greater boost from this all-round wonder food.

NUTRIENTS

Beta-carotene, folic acid, vitamin C;
calcium, magnesium, manganese,
phosphorus, potassium, sodium

ENERGY	★★★★☆
DETOX	★☆☆☆☆
IMMUNITY	★★★★☆
DIGESTION	★★★☆☆
SKIN	★★☆☆☆

121 | pineapple basic

½ pineapple
1 apple
3 carrots
1 stick celery

As long as you have the actual pineapple, this is a simple mixture of ingredients you're likely to have in your fruit bowl and refrigerator, and one which turns out a delicious morning juice.

NUTRIENTS

Beta-carotene, folic acid, vitamin C;
calcium, magnesium, manganese,
phosphorus, potassium, sodium,
sulphur

ENERGY	★★★★☆
DETOX	★★★★☆
IMMUNITY	★★★★☆
DIGESTION	★★★★☆
SKIN	★★★☆☆

122 | muddy pine

1 pineapple
1 teaspoon spirulina powder

The tangy, strong taste of the pineapple easily
carries the earthy goodness of the spirulina. Best
to shake a bit of the juice with the spirulina in a
jar and then mix it all up to avoid getting lumps
of green powder.

NUTRIENTS

Beta-carotene, folic acid, vitamins B1,	ENERGY	★★★★★
B3, B5, B6 and C; calcium, iron,	DETOX	★★★★★
magnesium, manganese, phosphorus,	IMMUNITY	★★★☆☆
potassium, sodium; protein,	DIGESTION	★★★★☆
essential fatty acids	SKIN	★★★★☆

123 | aniseed twist

$\frac{1}{2}$ pineapple
2 apples
$\frac{1}{2}$ fennel bulb

The fennel comes as an unexpected twist against the pineapple
and apple. A delicious afternoon pick-me-up.

NUTRIENTS

Beta-carotene, folic acid, vitamin C;	ENERGY	★★★★☆
calcium, magnesium, manganese,	DETOX	★★★☆☆
phosphorus, potassium, sodium,	IMMUNITY	★★★☆☆
sulphur	DIGESTION	★★★★☆
	SKIN	★★★☆☆

124 | bloody pineapple

½ pineapple
1 beet (beetroot)

Another mixture where the powerful taste of pineapple carries a flavour that some people find too earthy in other combinations.

NUTRIENTS

Beta-carotene, folic acid, vitamin C; calcium, magnesium, manganese, phosphorus, potassium, sodium

ENERGY	★★★★☆
DETOX	★★★★☆
IMMUNITY	★★★☆☆
DIGESTION	★★★★☆
SKIN	★★★★☆

125 | green pines

½ pineapple
3 sticks celery
1 large handful watercress

This is a very cleansing juice with rich, peppery undertones supplied by the watercress.

NUTRIENTS

Beta-carotene, folic acid, vitamin C, vitamin E; calcium, iron, magnesium, manganese, phosphorus, potassium, sodium, sulphur

ENERGY	★★★☆☆
DETOX	★★★★☆
IMMUNITY	★★★☆☆
DIGESTION	★★★☆☆
SKIN	★★★★☆

126 | digestaid

½ pineapple
1 thick slice white cabbage
1 inch (2.5 cm) ginger root
1 small bunch fresh mint

Pineapple contains bromelain (a natural substance that helps digestion), cabbage soothes the stomach lining and ginger calms the digestive tract – an all-round gut tonic.

NUTRIENTS

Beta-carotene, folic acid, vitamin C, vitamin E; calcium, magnesium, manganese, phosphorus, potassium, sodium

ENERGY	★★★☆☆
DETOX	★★★☆☆
IMMUNITY	★★☆☆☆
DIGESTION	★★★★★
SKIN	★★★☆☆

127 | joint aid

1 pineapple
2 inches (5 cm) ginger root
1 tablespoon flaxseed (linseed) oil

The bromelain in pineapple can help reduce inflammation, as can ginger
and the essential fatty acids in flax oil. Two inches of ginger is a pretty
hefty dose, so reduce it if you find it too strong.

NUTRIENTS

Beta-carotene, folic acid, vitamin C;
calcium, magnesium, manganese, phosphorus,
potassium, sodium; essential fatty acids

ENERGY	★★★★★
DETOX	★★★☆☆
IMMUNITY	★★★★★
DIGESTION	★★★★☆
SKIN	★★★★☆

128 | pineapple magic

½ pineapple
1 thick slice of melon
2 guavas

This exquisite combination of three flavoursome fruits
creates a creamy, magical taste which is also very rich
in immunity-boosting nutrients.

NUTRIENTS

Beta-carotene, folic acid,
vitamin B3, vitamin C; calcium,
magnesium, manganese, phosphorus,
potassium, sodium, sulphur

ENERGY	★★★★★
DETOX	★★☆☆☆
IMMUNITY	★★★★★
DIGESTION	★★★☆☆
SKIN	★★★☆☆

129 | what's up doc?

5 carrots

The original basic vegetable juice, this is pure orange, creamy and vibrant, and probably the most popular and palatable of all the solo vegetable juices.

NUTRIENTS

Beta-carotene, folic acid, vitamin C; calcium, magnesium, phosphorus, potassium, sodium, sulphur

ENERGY	★★★★☆
DETOX	★★★★☆
IMMUNITY	★★★★☆
DIGESTION	★★☆☆☆
SKIN	★★★★★

130 | easy morning

3 carrots
1 apple
$\frac{1}{2}$ orange
1 stick celery
$\frac{1}{2}$ inch (1 cm) ginger root

This is my absolute staple – when I'm not feeling any more adventurous, this is what pours daily from my juicer. It makes an invigorating start to any day.

NUTRIENTS

Beta-carotene, folic acid, vitamin C; calcium, magnesium, manganese, phosphorus, potassium, sodium, sulphur

ENERGY	★★★★☆
DETOX	★★★☆☆
IMMUNITY	★★★☆☆
DIGESTION	★★☆☆☆
SKIN	★★★☆☆

131 | apple basic

4 carrots
1 apple

Most refrigerators will house a couple of carrots and most fruit bowls an apple, so this is a good, basic standby for any morning.

NUTRIENTS

Beta-carotene, folic acid, vitamin C; calcium, magnesium, phosphorus, potassium, sodium, sulphur

ENERGY	★★★★★
DETOX	★★★☆☆
IMMUNITY	★★☆☆☆
DIGESTION	★★★☆☆
SKIN	★★★☆☆

132 | orange carrot

4 carrots
1 orange

Double-orange blast of colour and goodness — a great, basic blend for any morning.

NUTRIENTS

Beta-carotene, folic acid, vitamin C; calcium, magnesium, phosphorus, potassium, sodium, sulphur

ENERGY	★★★☆☆
DETOX	★★★☆☆
IMMUNITY	★★★☆☆
DIGESTION	★☆☆☆☆
SKIN	★★☆☆☆

133 | carrot cleanser

3 carrots
$\frac{1}{2}$ apple
$\frac{1}{2}$ orange
$\frac{1}{4}$ beet (beetroot)
1 stick celery
2 large kale leaves

Any juice using beet or kale can take some getting used to for the vegetable juice initiate, but once you've had it, you can fully appreciate its cleansing properties.

NUTRIENTS

Beta-carotene, folic acid, vitamins B3, B6 and C; calcium, iron, magnesium, manganese, phosphorus, potassium, sodium, sulphur

ENERGY	★★★☆☆
DETOX	★★★★★
IMMUNITY	★★★★☆
DIGESTION	★★★☆☆
SKIN	★★★☆☆

134 | carrot deep cleanser

3 carrots
$\frac{1}{2}$ apple
$\frac{1}{2}$ beet (beetroot)
1 stick celery
3 large kale leaves

If you are at all wary of having beet or kale juice, start with the Carrot
Cleanser before you graduate to this one.

NUTRIENTS

Beta-carotene, folic acid, vitamins B3,
B6 and C; calcium, iron, magnesium,
manganese, phosphorus, potassium,
sodium, sulphur

ENERGY	★★★☆☆
DETOX	★★★★★
IMMUNITY	★★★★☆
DIGESTION	★★★☆☆
SKIN	★★★☆☆

135 | carrot crunch

4 carrots
2 sticks celery
$\frac{1}{2}$ inch (1 cm) ginger root

Well, of course this isn't crunchy but if it weren't a juice it would certainly
get your jaw moving. An excellent contrasting blend of flavours.

NUTRIENTS

Beta-carotene, folic acid, vitamin C;
calcium, magnesium, phosphorus,
potassium, sodium, sulphur

ENERGY	★★★☆☆
DETOX	★★★☆☆
IMMUNITY	★★★★☆
DIGESTION	★★★☆☆
SKIN	★★★☆☆

136 | carrot digestif

4 carrots
$\frac{1}{4}$ pineapple
2 large white cabbage leaves

The beta-carotene in the carrots, combined with the particularly
soothing constituents of the other ingredients, makes this a great juice
for helping ease digestive problems.

NUTRIENTS

Beta-carotene, folic acid, vitamin C;
calcium, magnesium, manganese,
phosphorus, potassium, sodium, sulphur

ENERGY	★★★☆☆
DETOX	★★★☆☆
IMMUNITY	★☆☆☆☆
DIGESTION	★★★★★
SKIN	★★★☆☆

137 | carotene catapult

3 carrots
½ melon
1 slice watermelon
1 teaspoon spirulina

Beta-carotene is a crucial vitamin, which the body can convert to vitamin A.
It's needed for healthy immunity, skin, digestive tract, lungs and much more.
All of the ingredients in this tasty juice are excellent beta-carotene sources.

NUTRIENTS

Beta-carotene, folic acid, vitamins B1, B3,
B5, B6 and C; calcium, iron, magnesium,
phosphorus, potassium, sodium,
sulphur; protein, essential fatty acids

ENERGY	★★★★☆
DETOX	★★★☆☆
IMMUNITY	★★★★★
DIGESTION	★★★☆☆
SKIN	★★★★★

138 | sweet pepper

3 carrots
1 red bell pepper
1 yellow bell pepper

The sweetness of the carrots with bell peppers is remarkable and makes
this fresh drink a great introduction to vegetable-based juicing.

NUTRIENTS

Beta-carotene, folic acid, vitamin C;
calcium, magnesium, phosphorus,
potassium, sodium, sulphur

ENERGY	★★★☆☆
DETOX	★★☆☆☆
IMMUNITY	★★★★★
DIGESTION	★★☆☆☆
SKIN	★★★★☆

139 | breath freshener

4 medium carrots
1 handful parsley

This juice helps work on your breath from the inside, rather than just
washing out your mouth.

NUTRIENTS

Beta-carotene, folic acid, vitamin B3,
vitamin C; calcium, iron, magnesium,
phosphorus, potassium, sodium, sulphur

ENERGY	★★★★☆
DETOX	★★★☆☆
IMMUNITY	★★★★☆
DIGESTION	★★★★☆
SKIN	★★★★☆

140 | veggie carotene catapult

3 carrots
1 red bell pepper
1 spear broccoli
½ sweet potato

Superbly rich in anti-ageing
and cancer-protective carotenes
– and it tastes good.

NUTRIENTS

Beta-carotene, folic acid, vitamins C,
B5 and E; calcium, magnesium,
phosphorus, potassium, sodium,
sulphur

ENERGY   ★★★★☆
DETOX   ★★★☆☆
IMMUNITY   ★★★★★
DIGESTION   ★★★☆☆
SKIN   ★★★★★

141 | cold war

4 carrots
1 orange
½ inch (1 cm) ginger root
2 cloves garlic

The garlic in here is purely for therapeutic use – to give your immune
system a powerful punch in the face of a cold or any other infection.
It's a brave person who can stomach it on any normal morning, let
alone the breath you're likely to have afterwards. If your chest is feeling
congested, you could add half an onion.

NUTRIENTS

Beta-carotene, folic acid, vitamin C;   ENERGY   ★★★☆☆
calcium, magnesium, phosphorus,   DETOX   ★★☆☆☆
potassium, sodium, sulphur   IMMUNITY   ★★★★★
                                           DIGESTION   ★★☆☆☆
                                           SKIN   ★★★★☆

142 | sharp carrot

4 carrots
2 sticks celery
1 lime
1 small bunch fresh mint

This one has a fantastic bite from the lime, nicely lifted by the salty celery and hint of mint.

NUTRIENTS

Beta-carotene, folic acid, vitamin C; calcium, magnesium, phosphorus, potassium, sodium, sulphur

ENERGY	★★★★☆
DETOX	★★★☆☆
IMMUNITY	★★★☆☆
DIGESTION	★★★☆☆
SKIN	★★★☆☆

143 | minty carrot

3 carrots
1 apple
1 stick celery
1 small bunch fresh mint

A creamy, orange-coloured juice that could almost be pure fruit, it's so sweet, but the celery gives it a different turn.

NUTRIENTS

Beta-carotene, folic acid, vitamin C; calcium, magnesium, manganese, phosphorus, potassium, sodium, sulphur

ENERGY	★★★☆☆
DETOX	★★★☆☆
IMMUNITY	★★★★☆
DIGESTION	★★☆☆☆
SKIN	★★★☆☆

144 | carrot salad

3 carrots
2 tomatoes
2 sticks celery
½ lime

A fantastic blend of vegetable juices – makes you wonder why you would ever buy juice in a carton.

NUTRIENTS

Beta-carotene, biotin, folic acid, vitamin C; calcium, magnesium, phosphorus, potassium, sodium, sulphur

ENERGY	★★★☆☆
DETOX	★★☆☆☆
IMMUNITY	★★★☆☆
DIGESTION	★☆☆☆☆
SKIN	★★★★☆

145 | carrot lift

4 carrots
2 sticks celery
1 small bunch fresh parsley
$\frac{1}{2}$ lemon

A very refreshing combination – the creamy, sweet carrot offset by
the other ingredients.

NUTRIENTS

Beta-carotene, folic acid, vitamin B3,
vitamin C; calcium, iron, magnesium,
phosphorus, potassium, sodium, sulphur

ENERGY	★★★★☆
DETOX	★★★☆☆
IMMUNITY	★★★☆☆
DIGESTION	★★★☆☆
SKIN	★★★☆☆

146 | bloody carrot

3 carrots
1 beet (beetroot)
2 sticks celery
$\frac{1}{2}$ lime

A doubly rooty combination of sweetness lifted by the celery and
lime – wonderfully cleansing and fortifying.

NUTRIENTS

Beta-carotene, folic acid, vitamin C;
calcium, magnesium, manganese,
phosphorus, potassium, sodium,
sulphur

ENERGY	★★★☆☆
DETOX	★★★★☆
IMMUNITY	★★★★☆
DIGESTION	★★☆☆☆
SKIN	★★★★☆

147 | green hit

3 carrots
2 sticks celery
1 bunch watercress
1 large handful spinach

This is another very cleansing combination with earthy, grassy undertones.

NUTRIENTS

Beta-carotene, folic acid, vitamins B3,
C and E; calcium, iron, magnesium,
manganese, phosphorus, potassium,
sodium, sulphur

ENERGY	★★☆☆☆
DETOX	★★★☆☆
IMMUNITY	★★★☆☆
DIGESTION	★☆☆☆☆
SKIN	★★★☆☆

148 | carrot cooler

3 carrots
$\frac{1}{2}$ long cucumber
$\frac{1}{2}$ lime

Just the idea of cucumber is refreshing, let alone when you're drinking the juice, and it contrasts wonderfully well with the carrot.

NUTRIENTS

Beta-carotene, folic acid, vitamin C; calcium, magnesium, phosphorus, potassium, sodium, sulphur

ENERGY	★★★★☆
DETOX	★★★☆☆
IMMUNITY	★★★☆☆
DIGESTION	★☆☆☆☆
SKIN	★★★★☆

149 | florida carrot

3 carrots
$\frac{1}{2}$ grapefruit
1 orange
1 small handful mint leaves

The tang of the citrus complements the sweetness of the carrots perfectly.

NUTRIENTS

Beta-carotene, folic acid, vitamin C; calcium, magnesium, phosphorus, potassium, sodium, sulphur

ENERGY	★★★★☆
DETOX	★★☆☆☆
IMMUNITY	★★★★★
DIGESTION	★☆☆☆☆
SKIN	★★★☆☆

150 | chlorophyll carrot

4 carrots
1 orange
1 bunch fresh parsley

A surprisingly good combination and the high chlorophyll content of the parsley is wonderfully cleansing.

NUTRIENTS

Beta-carotene, folic acid, vitamin B3, vitamin C; calcium, iron, magnesium, phosphorus, potassium, sodium, sulphur

ENERGY	★★★★☆
DETOX	★★★★☆
IMMUNITY	★★★★☆
DIGESTION	★☆☆☆☆
SKIN	★★★★☆

151 | carrot tang

3 carrots
1 grapefruit
½ inch (1 cm) ginger root

I love the tang of the grapefruit tempered by the creamy carrot and then lifted by the zing of ginger – altogether an uplifting combination.

NUTRIENTS

Beta-carotene, folic acid, vitamin C; calcium, magnesium, phosphorus, potassium, sodium, sulphur

ENERGY	★★★★☆
DETOX	★★☆☆☆
IMMUNITY	★★★★☆
DIGESTION	★☆☆☆☆
SKIN	★★★☆☆

152 | triple orange

3 carrots
1 orange
½ melon

If you get the orange-fleshed variety of melon you get a threesome of orange and an explosion of tastes and a powerful beta-carotene hit.

NUTRIENTS

Beta-carotene, folic acid, vitamin C; calcium, magnesium, phosphorus, potassium, sodium, sulphur

ENERGY	★★★★★
DETOX	★★☆☆☆
IMMUNITY	★★★★★
DIGESTION	★☆☆☆☆
SKIN	★★★★☆

153 | capple zing

4 carrots
1 apple
½ inch (1 cm) ginger root
½ lime

Uplifting and fresh on the palate. This is a wonderful morning combination – very refreshing to awaken your tastebuds for the day.

NUTRIENTS

Beta-carotene, folic acid, vitamin C; calcium, magnesium, phosphorus, potassium, sodium, sulphur

ENERGY	★★★☆☆
DETOX	★★☆☆☆
IMMUNITY	★★★☆☆
DIGESTION	★☆☆☆☆
SKIN	★★☆☆☆

154 | capple kiwi

3 carrots
1 apple
2 kiwis

Kiwis can often be a bit soft to juice – choose firm ones and you'll
get a delicious green juice. A crisp apple such as Discovery goes
particularly well here.

NUTRIENTS

Beta-carotene, folic acid, vitamin C;
calcium, magnesium, phosphorus,
potassium, sodium, sulphur

ENERGY	★★★★★
DETOX	★★★☆☆
IMMUNITY	★★★★☆
DIGESTION	★★☆☆☆
SKIN	★★★★☆

155 | capple and black

4 carrots
1 apple
1 handful blackcurrants

That traditional favourite of apple and blackcurrant mixed with
creamy, sweet carrots makes a great combination.

NUTRIENTS

Beta-carotene, biotin, folic acid,
vitamin C, vitamin E; calcium,
magnesium, manganese, phosphorus,
potassium, sodium, sulphur

ENERGY	★★★☆☆
DETOX	★★☆☆☆
IMMUNITY	★★★★☆
DIGESTION	★☆☆☆☆
SKIN	★★★☆☆

156 | carrot jointaid

3 carrots
$\frac{1}{2}$ pineapple
1 inch (2.5 cm) ginger root
1 dessertspoon flaxseed (linseed) oil

A great combination of antioxidants and essential fats to help
soothe joints, plus pineapple and ginger which have been shown
to be anti-inflammatory and are good for problems such as asthma.

NUTRIENTS

Beta-carotene, folic acid, vitamin C;
calcium, magnesium, manganese,
phosphorus, potassium, sodium,
sulphur; essential fatty acids

ENERGY	★★★☆☆
DETOX	★★★☆☆
IMMUNITY	★★★☆☆
DIGESTION	★★★☆☆
SKIN	★★☆☆☆

157 | cool 'n' creamy

1 cucumber
4 carrots

Each of these juices brings out the best in the other. You'll be surprised at just how much flavour you can extract from juicing a cucumber, and how delicious it is.

NUTRIENTS

Beta-carotene, folic acid, vitamin C;
calcium, magnesium, phosphorus,
potassium, sodium, sulphur

ENERGY	★★☆☆☆
DETOX	★★★☆☆
IMMUNITY	★★☆☆☆
DIGESTION	★☆☆☆☆
SKIN	★★☆☆☆

158 | cool 'n' pale

1 cucumber
2 apples

A dreamy shade of green, with a taste to match – this refreshing combination of two highly juicy ingredients is very cleansing on the palate.

NUTRIENTS

Beta-carotene, folic acid,
vitamin C; calcium, magnesium,
phosphorus, potassium, sulphur

ENERGY	★★★☆☆
DETOX	★★★★☆
IMMUNITY	★★☆☆☆
DIGESTION	★★★☆☆
SKIN	★★★☆☆

159 | cucumber refresher

1 cucumber
2 pears

Another delicate mix of pale green with two subtly flavoured ingredients
blending to form a refreshing, cleansing juice.

NUTRIENTS

Beta-carotene, folic acid, vitamin C;
calcium, magnesium, phosphorus,
potassium, sulphur

ENERGY	★★★☆☆
DETOX	★★★★☆
IMMUNITY	★★☆☆☆
DIGESTION	★★★☆☆
SKIN	★★★☆☆

160 | apple cooler

1 cucumber
2 apples
4 sprigs fresh mint
$\frac{1}{2}$ inch (1 cm) ginger root

A wonderful summer drink. You could even add a splash of ginger
ale or fizzy water for a non-alcoholic cocktail.

NUTRIENTS

Beta-carotene, folic acid, vitamin C;
calcium, magnesium, phosphorus,
potassium, sulphur

ENERGY	★★★☆☆
DETOX	★★★★☆
IMMUNITY	★★☆☆☆
DIGESTION	★★★☆☆
SKIN	★★★☆☆

161 | mellow melon

$\frac{3}{4}$ cucumber
$\frac{1}{2}$ melon
1 pear
2 sprigs mint

From the same family, cucumber and melon combine beautifully.
You can leave out the mint if you prefer.

NUTRIENTS

Beta-carotene, folic acid, vitamin C;
calcium, magnesium, phosphorus,
potassium, sodium, sulphur

ENERGY	★★★★☆
DETOX	★★★★☆
IMMUNITY	★★★☆☆
DIGESTION	★★★☆☆
SKIN	★★★☆☆

162 | water water everywhere

1 cucumber
1 thick slice watermelon

Two of the juiciest of nature's pickings blend to create a rich but
subtle flavour. A perfect summer thirst-quencher.

NUTRIENTS

Beta-carotene, folic acid, vitamin B5,
vitamin C; calcium, magnesium,
phosphorus, potassium, sodium

ENERGY	★★★★☆
DETOX	★★★★☆
IMMUNITY	★★★★☆
DIGESTION	★★☆☆☆
SKIN	★★★☆☆

163 | citrus cuke

1 cucumber
1 orange
1 grapefruit

Although the actual flavour of the cucumber gets a bit lost, its
watery freshness transforms the orange and grapefruit to a more
refreshing drink.

NUTRIENTS

Beta-carotene, folic acid, vitamin C;
calcium, magnesium, phosphorus,
potassium, sulphur

ENERGY	★★★★☆
DETOX	★★☆☆☆
IMMUNITY	★★★★☆
DIGESTION	☆☆☆☆☆
SKIN	★★★☆☆

164 | salad cooler

1 cucumber
3 tomatoes
1 small bunch fresh parsley
$\frac{1}{2}$ lemon

A great veggie cocktail which always reminds me of a fresh, tasty
Middle Eastern salad.

NUTRIENTS

Beta-carotene, biotin, folic acid,
vitamin B3, vitamin C; calcium, iron,
magnesium, phosphorus, potassium,
sodium, sulphur

ENERGY	★★☆☆☆
DETOX	★★★★☆
IMMUNITY	★★★☆☆
DIGESTION	★☆☆☆☆
SKIN	★★★★☆

165 | tropical cucumber

1 cucumber
2 guavas
1 apple

The rich, tangy, tropical taste of guavas
is toned down by the cucumber to form
an unusual cooling juice.

NUTRIENTS

Beta-carotene, folic acid, vitamin B3,
vitamin C; calcium, magnesium, phosphorus,
potassium, sodium, sulphur

ENERGY	★★★★☆
DETOX	★★★★☆
IMMUNITY	★★★★☆
DIGESTION	★★☆☆☆
SKIN	★★★★☆

166 | bloody cuke

1 cucumber
2 apples
1 beet (beetroot)

The richness of the beet is perfectly tempered by the cucumber
and sweetened by the apple in this colourful magenta juice.

NUTRIENTS

Beta-carotene, folic acid, vitamin C;
calcium, magnesium, phosphorus,
potassium, sodium, sulphur

ENERGY	★★★☆☆
DETOX	★★★★★
IMMUNITY	★★★☆☆
DIGESTION	★★★★☆
SKIN	★★★★☆

167 | green goddess

1 bunch fresh parsley
1 handful watercress
4 broccoli spears
$\frac{1}{2}$ pineapple

There had to be one juice with this name and this is it – anything with pineapple is good in my book.

NUTRIENTS
Beta-carotene, folic acid, vitamins B3,
B5, C and E; calcium, iron, magnesium,
phosphorus, potassium, sodium, sulphur

ENERGY	★★★☆☆
DETOX	★★★★★
IMMUNITY	★★☆☆☆
DIGESTION	★★★★☆
SKIN	★★★★☆

168 | green apple

8 spears broccoli
1 bunch parsley
3 apples

To counteract the strong-tasting green vegetables, it's best to use an apple variety with a strong flavour, such as Granny Smith, for this one.

NUTRIENTS
Beta-carotene, folic acid, vitamins B3,
B5 and C; calcium, iron, magnesium,
phosphorus, potassium, sodium, sulphur

ENERGY	★★☆☆☆
DETOX	★★★★★
IMMUNITY	★★★★☆
DIGESTION	★★★★☆
SKIN	★★★★☆

169 | green 'n' pear it

8 spears broccoli
3 sticks celery
2 pears

You may not wish to adulterate your pear with broccoli juice but believe me, it's a surprising winner.

NUTRIENTS
Beta-carotene, folic acid, vitamin B5,
vitamin C; calcium, magnesium,
phosphorus, potassium, sodium,
sulphur

ENERGY	★★★☆☆
DETOX	★★★★★
IMMUNITY	★★★★☆
DIGESTION	★★★★☆
SKIN	★★★★☆

170 | green citrus

2 handfuls spinach
2 sticks celery
2 oranges

The orange juice is so flavourful that it can carry pretty much anything,
even the powerful taste of iron-rich spinach.

NUTRIENTS

Beta-carotene, folic acid, vitamin B3,
vitamin C; calcium, iron, magnesium,
phosphorus, potassium, sodium, sulphur

ENERGY	★★★☆☆
DETOX	★★★☆☆
IMMUNITY	★★★★☆
DIGESTION	★☆☆☆☆
SKIN	★★★☆☆

171 | green grapefruit

8 broccoli spears
2 grapefruits

If anything is going to temper the strong, earthy taste of broccoli
juice and make it more palatable, it's going to be grapefruit.

NUTRIENTS

Beta-carotene, folic acid, vitamin B5,
vitamin C; calcium, magnesium,
phosphorus, potassium, sodium,
sulphur

ENERGY	★★★☆☆
DETOX	★★★★★
IMMUNITY	★★★★☆
DIGESTION	★☆☆☆☆
SKIN	★★★★☆

172 | green waldorf

5 large kale leaves
2 apples
2 sticks celery
1 dessertspoon flaxseed (linseed) oil

Well, not quite a Waldorf, but it tastes good and is super-healthy.
The flax brings an unusual dimension in taste, texture and health
properties to this cleansing juice.

NUTRIENTS

Beta-carotene, folic acid, vitamin B3,
vitamin C; calcium, iron, magnesium,
manganese, phosphorus, potassium,
sodium, sulphur

ENERGY	★★★☆☆
DETOX	★★★★☆
IMMUNITY	★★★☆☆
DIGESTION	★★★★☆
SKIN	★★★★☆

173 | sweet green melon

1 bunch parsley
$\frac{1}{4}$ white cabbage
$\frac{1}{2}$ long cucumber
$\frac{1}{2}$ melon

The green in this doesn't just belong to the melon – it's a cleansing punch, tempered by cucumber.

NUTRIENTS

Beta-carotene, folic acid, vitamins B3,
C and E; calcium, iron, magnesium,
phosphorus, potassium, sodium,
sulphur

ENERGY	★★★☆☆
DETOX	★★★★☆
IMMUNITY	★★★☆☆
DIGESTION	★★★★★
SKIN	★★★★☆

174 | green lullaby

$\frac{1}{2}$ lettuce
2 apples
$\frac{1}{2}$ lime
1 small handful spinach

Lettuces contain substances which act as mild sedatives, so this one should help send you into the land of nod.

NUTRIENTS

Beta-carotene, folic acid, vitamin B3,
vitamin C; calcium, iron, magnesium,
phosphorus, potassium, sodium, sulphur

ENERGY	★☆☆☆☆
DETOX	★★★☆☆
IMMUNITY	★★★☆☆
DIGESTION	☆☆☆☆☆
SKIN	★★☆☆☆

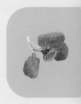

175 | super defender

5 large kale leaves
3 carrots
1 orange

Kale, orange and carrot – muddy to look at, magnificent to taste.

NUTRIENTS

Beta-carotene, folic acid, vitamin B3,
vitamin C; calcium, iron, magnesium,
manganese, phosphorus, potassium,
sodium, sulphur

ENERGY	★★★☆☆
DETOX	★★★★☆
IMMUNITY	★★★★★
DIGESTION	☆☆☆☆☆
SKIN	★★★★☆

176 | grape & green

4 large kale leaves
2 handfuls spinach
2 sticks celery
1 grapefruit

The tangy grapefruit and salty celery cut right through the earthy
taste of the greens in this rejuvenating juice.

NUTRIENTS

Beta-carotene, folic acid, vitamin C;
calcium, magnesium, manganese,
phosphorus, potassium, sodium,
sulphur

ENERGY	★★☆☆☆
DETOX	★★★★☆
IMMUNITY	★★★★☆
DIGESTION	★★☆☆☆
SKIN	★★★★☆

177 | creamy green

1 bunch parsley
1 handful watercress
4 carrots
1 lime

The sweet, creamy carrot juice carries the greens very well,
and the lime gives it a good, sharp kick.

NUTRIENTS

Beta-carotene, folic acid, vitamins B3,
C and E; calcium, iron, magnesium,
phosphorus, potassium, sodium,
sulphur

ENERGY	★★★☆☆
DETOX	★★★★★
IMMUNITY	★★★★★
DIGESTION	★★★☆☆
SKIN	★★★★☆

178 | red & green

1 bunch parsley
1 lemon
5 tomatoes

This is a fantastically cleansing juice, and another one with
Middle Eastern salad undertones.

NUTRIENTS

Beta-carotene, biotin, folic acid,
vitamin B3, vitamin C; calcium, iron,
magnesium, phosphorus, potassium,
sodium, sulphur

ENERGY	★★★☆☆
DETOX	★★★★☆
IMMUNITY	★★★★☆
DIGESTION	★☆☆☆☆
SKIN	★★★★☆

179 | beet basic

2 beets (beetroot)
2 carrots
1 apple
1 orange
1 sticks celery
$\frac{1}{2}$ inch (1 cm) ginger root

If I have beets in the refrigerator, this is one of my standard morning
juices. It's a supreme energy-lifting, cleansing and immune-boosting blend.

NUTRIENTS

Beta-carotene, folic acid, vitamin C;
calcium, magnesium, phosphorus,
potassium, sodium, sulphur

ENERGY	★★★★☆
DETOX	★★★★☆
IMMUNITY	★★★★☆
DIGESTION	★★★☆☆
SKIN	★★★★☆

180 | beetles

2 beets (beetroot)
2 apples
3 sticks celery

Another great combination
of beet and fruit, enhanced
by the celery.

NUTRIENTS

Beta-carotene, folic acid, vitamin C;
calcium, magnesium, phosphorus,
potassium, sodium, sulphur

ENERGY	★★★★☆
DETOX	★★★★★
IMMUNITY	★★★☆☆
DIGESTION	★★★☆☆
SKIN	★★★★☆

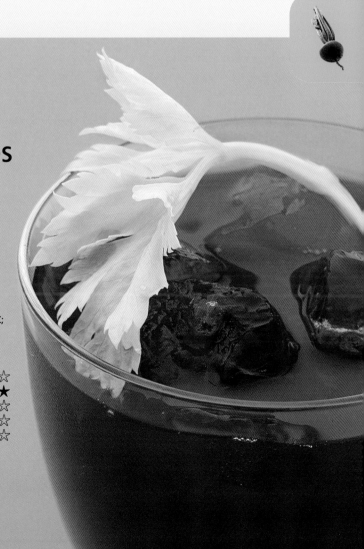

181 | blood 'n' grape

2 beets (beetroot)
1 grapefruit
2 sticks celery

Grapefruit carries that earthy, sweet beet well and both are lifted by
the salty celery – a convincing introduction to beet, if you need one.

NUTRIENTS

Beta-carotene, folic acid, vitamin C;
calcium, magnesium, phosphorus,
potassium, sodium, sulphur

ENERGY	★★★★☆
DETOX	★★★★☆
IMMUNITY	★★★★☆
DIGESTION	★★☆☆☆
SKIN	★★★★☆

182 | blood & carrots

2 beets (beetroot)
2 oranges (ideally blood oranges)
4 carrots

Blood oranges or not, this sumptuous juice is going to be a rich,
purple colour, swirling with the creamy orange from the carrots.

NUTRIENTS

Beta-carotene, folic acid, vitamin C;
calcium, magnesium, phosphorus,
potassium, sodium, sulphur

ENERGY	★★★★☆
DETOX	★★★☆☆
IMMUNITY	★★★★★
DIGESTION	★★☆☆☆
SKIN	★★★★☆

183 | rooty pear

3 parsnips
3 pears
1 lime

A blend of very delicate, sweet flavours, sharpened by the lime.

NUTRIENTS

Beta-carotene, folic acid, vitamin C;
calcium, magnesium, phosphorus,
potassium, sodium, sulphur

ENERGY	★★★★☆
DETOX	★★☆☆☆
IMMUNITY	★★★☆☆
DIGESTION	★☆☆☆☆
SKIN	★★☆☆☆

184 | apples & neeps

3 parsnips
3 apples
$\frac{1}{2}$ lime
3 sprigs mint

If you're at all hesitant to try root vegetable juice, this is a good one
to start with. Add more lime if you want to give it more tang.

NUTRIENTS

Beta-carotene, folic acid, vitamin C;
calcium, magnesium, phosphorus,
potassium, sodium, sulphur

ENERGY	★★★★☆
DETOX	★★★☆☆
IMMUNITY	★★★☆☆
DIGESTION	★★☆☆☆
SKIN	★★☆☆☆

185 | carotene kick

1 sweet potato
$\frac{1}{2}$ melon
3 carrots

Sweet potatoes are a delicious, rich source of carotene, as are the other
ingredients in this vibrant orange drink.

NUTRIENTS

Beta-carotene, folic acid, vitamin C,
vitamin E; calcium, magnesium, phosphorus,
potassium, sodium, sulphur

ENERGY	★★★★★
DETOX	★★★☆☆
IMMUNITY	★★★★★
DIGESTION	★★★☆☆
SKIN	★★★★★

186 | pineroot

1 sweet potato
1 carrot
$\frac{1}{2}$ pineapple

The root vegetables tone down the tangy pineapple for a sweet drink.

NUTRIENTS

Beta-carotene, folic acid, vitamin C,
vitamin E; calcium, magnesium, manganese,
phosphorus, potassium, sodium, sulphur

ENERGY	★★★★★
DETOX	★★★☆☆
IMMUNITY	★★★★★
DIGESTION	★★★★★
SKIN	★★★★☆

187 | pure tomato

8 tomatoes
salt, pepper, Tobasco,
Worcestershire Sauce to taste

One of the few vegetable juices that is wonderful unadulterated. You can
always add a squeeze of lemon juice if you're not into the pure stuff.

NUTRIENTS

Beta-carotene, biotin, folic acid,
vitamin C; calcium, magnesium,
phosphorus, potassium, sodium,
sulphur

ENERGY	★★★★☆
DETOX	★★☆☆☆
IMMUNITY	★★★★☆
DIGESTION	☆☆☆☆☆
SKIN	★★★★☆

188 | ginger tom

6 tomatoes
2 sticks celery
1 inch (2.5 cm) ginger root

Celery is probably my favourite juice to combine with tomatoes – the
light saltiness taking the edge off the richer tomato and the ginger in
this one gives it all a sharp lift. You can be even more daring with the
amount of ginger you use if you like.

NUTRIENTS

Beta-carotene, biotin, folic acid,
vitamin C; calcium, magnesium,
manganese, phosphorus, potassium,
sodium, sulphur

ENERGY	★★★★☆
DETOX	★★☆☆☆
IMMUNITY	★★★★☆
DIGESTION	★☆☆☆☆
SKIN	★★★★☆

189 | tabouleh

6 tomatoes
1 large bunch parsley
1 lemon
salt and pepper to taste

If you are a fan of tomato and parsley salad or tabouleh, you'll love this
one. Season with some salt and pepper.

NUTRIENTS

Beta-carotene, biotin, folic acid,
vitamin B3, vitamin C; calcium, iron,
magnesium, phosphorus, potassium,
sodium, sulphur

ENERGY	★★★☆☆
DETOX	★★★☆☆
IMMUNITY	★★★★☆
DIGESTION	★☆☆☆☆
SKIN	★★★★☆

190 | tomato bell

6 tomatoes
2 bell peppers
1 stick celery
$\frac{1}{2}$ lemon
salt, pepper, Tobasco,
Worcestershire Sauce to taste

I'd only use red or yellow peppers for this as
the green ones tend to take over the other
flavours. Season it well once you've made
the juice, sit back and sip it slowly, nibbling
from a bowl of potato chips, nuts and olives.

NUTRIENTS
Beta-carotene, biotin, folic acid, vitamin B3,
vitamin C; calcium, iron, magnesium,
phosphorus, potassium, sodium, sulphur

ENERGY	★★★★☆
DETOX	★★☆☆☆
IMMUNITY	★★★★☆
DIGESTION	☆☆☆☆☆
SKIN	★★★☆☆

191 | peppery tom

6 tomatoes
1 large bunch watercress
1 stick celery

The watercress in this acts as a seasoning all to itself, and the celery
lightens the rich taste of the tomatoes.

NUTRIENTS
Beta-carotene, biotin, folic acid,
vitamin C, vitamin E; calcium,
iron, magnesium, phosphorus,
potassium, sodium, sulphur

ENERGY	★★★★☆
DETOX	★★★★☆
IMMUNITY	★★★★☆
DIGESTION	★☆☆☆☆
SKIN	★★★★☆

192 | sweet 'n' fresh

6 tomatoes
1 red bell pepper
1 stick celery
1 large bunch parsley

The wonderful sweetness of the tomatoes and peppers is heightened
by the salty celery and freshened further by the parsley.

NUTRIENTS

Beta-carotene, biotin, folic acid,
vitamin B3, vitamin C; calcium, iron,
magnesium, manganese, phosphorus,
potassium, sodium, sulphur

ENERGY	★★★★☆
DETOX	★★★☆☆
IMMUNITY	★★★★☆
DIGESTION	★☆☆☆☆
SKIN	★★★★☆

193 | classic combo

6 tomatoes
3 carrots
1 lime
1 small bunch mint

The two most popular and palatable of the vegetable juices combined
with a lift from the mint and lime.

NUTRIENTS

Beta-carotene, biotin, folic acid,
vitamin C; calcium, magnesium,
phosphorus, potassium, sodium,
sulphur

ENERGY	★★★★☆
DETOX	★★★☆☆
IMMUNITY	★★★★☆
DIGESTION	★☆☆☆☆
SKIN	★★★★☆

194 | green tomatoes

4 tomatoes
½ long cucumber
1 large handful spinach leaves
4 broccoli spears

Not fried like at the Whistlestop Café, but blended with greens for a
deep cleansing juice. The earthy, green taste of the spinach and broccoli
is nicely hidden by the other ingredients.

NUTRIENTS

Beta-carotene, biotin, folic acid,
vitamin B3, vitamin C; calcium, iron,
magnesium, phosphorus, potassium,
sodium, sulphur

ENERGY	★★★☆☆
DETOX	★★★★☆
IMMUNITY	★★★☆☆
DIGESTION	☆☆☆☆☆
SKIN	★★☆☆☆

195 | root tomato

4 tomatoes
4 carrots
1 handful radishes
salt, pepper and a squeeze of lemon to taste

No, not a tomato modified to grow underground, but a blend with
wonderfully contrasting vegetables that do.

NUTRIENTS

Beta-carotene, biotin, folic acid,
vitamin C; calcium, magnesium,
phosphorus, potassium, sodium,
sulphur

ENERGY	★★★★☆
DETOX	★★☆☆☆
IMMUNITY	★★★★☆
DIGESTION	★☆☆☆☆
SKIN	★★★★☆

196 | tricolore

6 tomatoes
2 parsnips
2 sticks celery
1 small handful of basil leaves

No mozzarella in here, but a red, white and green combination
anyway, and the unusual touch from the basil will transport you
straight to Italy.

NUTRIENTS

Beta-carotene, biotin, folic acid,
vitamin C; calcium, magnesium,
manganese, phosphorus, potassium,
sodium, sulphur

ENERGY	★★★★☆
DETOX	★★★☆☆
IMMUNITY	★★★☆☆
DIGESTION	★☆☆☆☆
SKIN	★★★☆☆

197 | red tomato

6 tomatoes
1 beet (beetroot)
1 lemon

You may have found by now that unlike tomato juice from a carton,
the stuff you make at home is not red but pink, so the title may not
be stating the obvious. Here it's the inimitable velvet red-purple of
the beet that colours the juice.

NUTRIENTS

Beta-carotene, biotin, folic acid,
vitamin C; calcium, magnesium,
phosphorus, potassium, sodium,
sulphur

ENERGY	★★★★☆
DETOX	★★★★☆
IMMUNITY	★★★★★
DIGESTION	☆☆☆☆☆
SKIN	★★★☆☆

198 | black mud

5 tomatoes
1 beet (beetroot)
4 large kale leaves
1 lime

Not the most appetizing colour but it sure makes up for that in taste and some unbeatable health benefits.

NUTRIENTS

Beta-carotene, biotin, folic acid,
vitamin B3, vitamin C; calcium, iron,
magnesium, manganese, phosphorus,
potassium, sodium, sulphur

ENERGY	★★★★☆
DETOX	★★★★★
IMMUNITY	★★★★★
DIGESTION	★☆☆☆☆
SKIN	★★★☆☆

199 | cool as a tomato

5 tomatoes
½ long cucumber
salt, pepper, Tobasco, Worcestershire Sauce to taste

As always with juices containing cucumber, this is a light, refreshing blend and another one which goes down well with some seasoning.

NUTRIENTS

Beta-carotene, biotin, folic acid,
vitamin C; calcium, magnesium,
phosphorus, potassium, sodium,
sulphur

ENERGY	★★★☆☆
DETOX	★★☆☆☆
IMMUNITY	★★★☆☆
DIGESTION	☆☆☆☆☆
SKIN	★★☆☆☆

200 | tomato cocktail

6 tomatoes
¼ long cucumber
½ inch (1 cm) ginger root
1 small bunch mint leaves
1 lime

The cucumber is added to refresh, and then the mint, lime and ginger to take it all onto an even higher plane.

NUTRIENTS

Beta-carotene, biotin, folic acid,
vitamin C; calcium, magnesium,
phosphorus, potassium, sodium,
sulphur

ENERGY	★★★☆☆
DETOX	★★☆☆☆
IMMUNITY	★★★☆☆
DIGESTION	★☆☆☆☆
SKIN	★★☆☆☆

201 | classic & green

6 tomatoes
3 carrots
1 large handful spinach

Classic with an earthy, green undertone,
this juice is particularly good for the
immune system as it's packed with carotenes.

NUTRIENTS

Beta-carotene, biotin, folic acid,
vitamin B3, vitamin C; calcium,
iron, magnesium, phosphorus,
potassium, sodium, sulphur

ENERGY	★★★★☆
DETOX	★★★☆☆
IMMUNITY	★★★★★
DIGESTION	☆☆☆☆☆
SKIN	★★★★☆

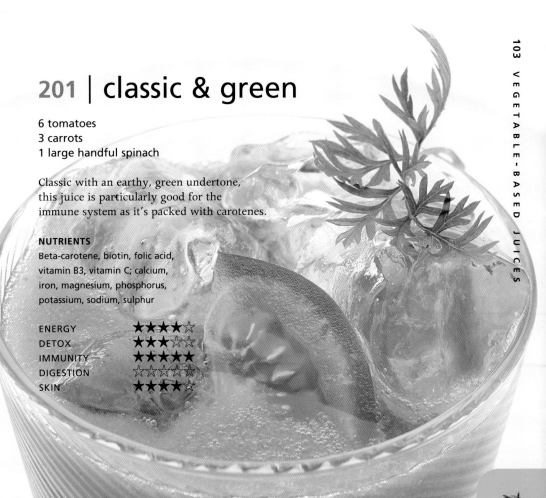

202 | old favourites

4 tomatoes
1 orange
2 carrots

Three of the most popular individual juices rolled into one to create
an interesting tasting juice that is great for your immunity.

NUTRIENTS

Beta-carotene, biotin, folic acid,
vitamin C; calcium, magnesium,
phosphorus, potassium, sodium,
sulphur

ENERGY	★★★★☆
DETOX	★★☆☆☆
IMMUNITY	★★★★★
DIGESTION	☆☆☆☆☆
SKIN	★★★★☆

203 | tomorange

4 tomatoes
2 oranges

Probably the only combination of tomato juice with fruit that
I think really works – very refreshing and very good for you.

NUTRIENTS

Beta-carotene, biotin, folic acid,
vitamin C; calcium, magnesium,
phosphorus, potassium, sodium,
sulphur

ENERGY	★★★★☆
DETOX	★★☆☆☆
IMMUNITY	★★★★★
DIGESTION	☆☆☆☆☆
SKIN	★★★☆☆

204 | tomorange fresh

4 tomatoes
2 oranges
1 small handful fresh mint leaves

Just as above with a hint of mint that takes it up a notch in the
refreshing stakes. A great immune-booster as well.

NUTRIENTS

Beta-carotene, biotin, folic acid,
vitamin C; calcium, magnesium,
phosphorus, potassium, sodium,
sulphur

ENERGY	★★★★☆
DETOX	★★☆☆☆
IMMUNITY	★★★★★
DIGESTION	★☆☆☆☆
SKIN	★★★☆☆

205 | creamy crunch

4 sticks celery
3 carrots

Each of these juices brings out the best in the other.

NUTRIENTS

Beta-carotene, folic acid, vitamin C;
calcium, magnesium, manganese,
phosphorus, potassium, sodium,
sulphur

ENERGY	★★★☆☆
DETOX	★★★★☆
IMMUNITY	★★★☆☆
DIGESTION	★★★☆☆
SKIN	★★★☆☆

206 | cool 'n' pale II

4 sticks celery
2 apples

A dreamy shade of green, with a taste to match. Discovery apples
make an ideal partner for the celery in this one.

NUTRIENTS

Beta-carotene, folic acid, vitamin C;
calcium, magnesium, manganese,
phosphorus, potassium, sodium,
sulphur

ENERGY	★★☆☆☆
DETOX	★★★☆☆
IMMUNITY	★★☆☆☆
DIGESTION	★★★☆☆
SKIN	★★☆☆☆

207 | savoury fruit

3 sticks celery
1 apple
1 orange

The celery here lifts the flavours of the fruit juices.

NUTRIENTS

Beta-carotene, folic acid, vitamin C;
calcium, magnesium, manganese,
phosphorus, potassium, sodium,
sulphur

ENERGY	★★★☆☆
DETOX	★★★☆☆
IMMUNITY	★★★☆☆
DIGESTION	★☆☆☆☆
SKIN	★★☆☆☆

208 | delicate pale

4 sticks celery
2 pears

Because pears tend to have a more delicate
flavour than apples, this one is even more
subtle than Cool 'n' Pale II (see p.105), but is
just as refreshing.

NUTRIENTS
Beta-carotene, folic acid, vitamin C;
calcium, magnesium, phosphorus,
potassium, sodium, sulphur

ENERGY	★★★☆☆
DETOX	★★★★☆
IMMUNITY	★★☆☆☆
DIGESTION	★★★☆☆
SKIN	★★☆☆☆

209 | crunch morning favourite

3 sticks celery
1 grapefruit
$\frac{1}{2}$ inch (1 cm) ginger root

One of a few standard morning favourites to come out of my fruit bowl
and refrigerator. Grapefruit always seems to go well with vegetable juices.

NUTRIENTS
Beta-carotene, folic acid, vitamin C;
calcium, magnesium, manganese,
phosphorus, potassium, sodium,
sulphur

ENERGY	★★☆☆☆
DETOX	★★★☆☆
IMMUNITY	★★★☆☆
DIGESTION	★☆☆☆☆
SKIN	★★☆☆☆

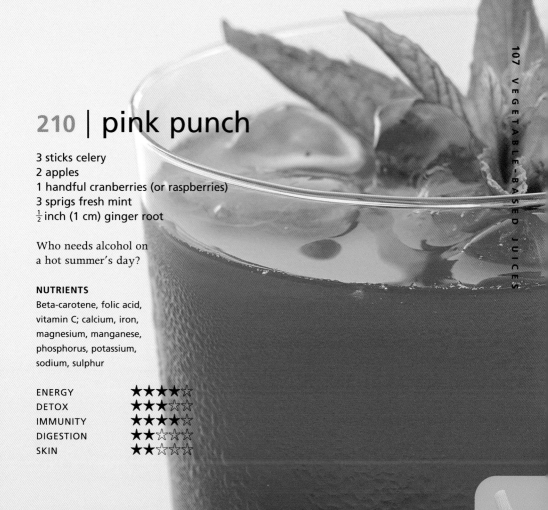

210 | pink punch

3 sticks celery
2 apples
1 handful cranberries (or raspberries)
3 sprigs fresh mint
$\frac{1}{2}$ inch (1 cm) ginger root

Who needs alcohol on
a hot summer's day?

NUTRIENTS

Beta-carotene, folic acid,
vitamin C; calcium, iron,
magnesium, manganese,
phosphorus, potassium,
sodium, sulphur

ENERGY	★★★★☆
DETOX	★★★☆☆
IMMUNITY	★★★★☆
DIGESTION	★★☆☆☆
SKIN	★★☆☆☆

211 | celery jointaid

3 sticks celery
$\frac{1}{2}$ pineapple
1 inch (2.5 cm) ginger root
1 dessertspoon flaxseed (linseed) oil

A combination of minerals, antioxidants and essential fats to help
support healthy joints, this fresh juice also offers the anti-inflammatory
properties of pineapple and ginger.

NUTRIENTS

Beta-carotene, folic acid, vitamin C;
calcium, magnesium, manganese,
phosphorus, potassium, sodium,
sulphur; essential fatty acids

ENERGY	★★★★☆
DETOX	★★★★☆
IMMUNITY	★★★★★
DIGESTION	★★★★★
SKIN	★★★☆☆

212 | fresh crunch

4 sticks celery
1 apple
5 sprigs fresh mint
1 lime

A startling, fresh combination – use more lime if you fancy giving
it a sharper bite.

NUTRIENTS

Beta-carotene, folic acid, vitamin C;	ENERGY ★★☆☆☆
calcium, magnesium, manganese,	DETOX ★★★★☆
phosphorus, potassium, sodium,	IMMUNITY ★★★☆☆
sulphur	DIGESTION ★★☆☆☆
	SKIN ★★★☆☆

213 | salty sharp melon

3 sticks celery
½ melon
1 lime

Melon juice is so sweet and creamy – here the celery and lime lift
it to a sharper plane.

NUTRIENTS

Beta-carotene, folic acid, vitamin C;	ENERGY ★★★☆☆
calcium, magnesium, manganese,	DETOX ★★★☆☆
phosphorus, potassium, sodium,	IMMUNITY ★★★★☆
sulphur	DIGESTION ☆☆☆☆☆
	SKIN ★★★☆☆

214 | soft and sharp

3 sticks celery
2 pears
1 large bunch watercress

The sharp contrast between the pear and the watercress goes well
with the fresh, salty celery in this pretty, green drink.

NUTRIENTS

Beta-carotene, folic acid, vitamin C,	ENERGY ★★☆☆☆
vitamin E; calcium, iron, magnesium,	DETOX ★★★★★
phosphorus, potassium, sodium,	IMMUNITY ★★★★☆
sulphur	DIGESTION ★★★☆☆
	SKIN ★★★☆☆

215 | grape crunch

4 sticks celery
1 large bunch seedless grapes (about 50)

There's something about the sweetness of grapes that goes fantastically well with celery. Use either green or red grapes, although red are richer in antioxidants.

NUTRIENTS

Folic acid, vitamin C, vitamin E;
calcium, manganese, phosphorus,
potassium, sodium, sulphur

ENERGY	★★★★☆
DETOX	★★★★☆
IMMUNITY	★★★☆☆
DIGESTION	★★☆☆☆
SKIN	★★★☆☆

216 | tricolore cruncher

3 sticks celery
3 tomatoes
1 small bunch parsley
1 handful watercress
$\frac{1}{2}$ lemon

Fresh and cleansing – with a kick from the watercress and lemon, this is a delicious, salad-like combination.

NUTRIENTS

Beta-carotene, biotin, folic acid,
vitamins B3, C and E; calcium, iron,
magnesium, manganese, phosphorus,
potassium, sodium, sulphur

ENERGY	★★☆☆☆
DETOX	★★★★☆
IMMUNITY	★★★☆☆
DIGESTION	☆☆☆☆☆
SKIN	★★★★★

217 | take heart

4 sticks celery
1 apple
1 handful blackcurrants
½ inch (1 cm) ginger root
1 dessertspoon flaxseed (linseed) oil

Each of the ingredients in this bright juice has properties that can help support healthy blood pressure and blood vessels — and it tastes great.

NUTRIENTS

Beta-carotene, biotin, folic acid, vitamin C, vitamin E; calcium, magnesium, manganese, phosphorus, potassium, sodium, sulphur; essential fatty acids

ENERGY	★★★☆☆
DETOX	★★★★☆
IMMUNITY	★★★★☆
DIGESTION	★★☆☆☆
SKIN	★★★★☆

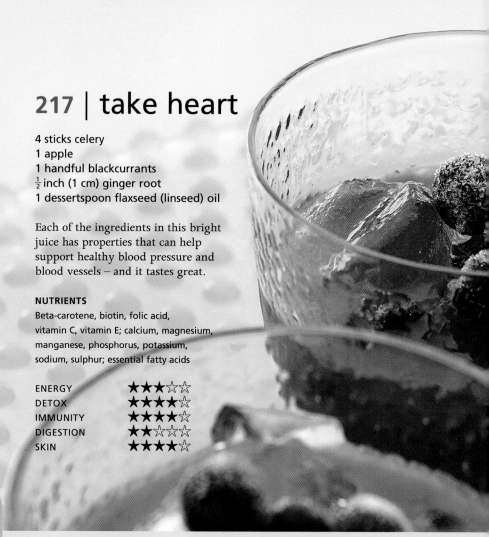

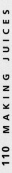

218 | chlorophyll crunch

3 sticks celery
3 carrots
1 bunch parsley

Creamy carrots, salty celery and perky parsley combine in this substantial drink that is a good detoxifier and all-round immune-boosting tonic. You really can taste the goodness.

NUTRIENTS

Beta-carotene, folic acid, vitamin B3, vitamin C; calcium, iron, magnesium, manganese, phosphorus, potassium, sodium, sulphur

ENERGY	★★☆☆☆
DETOX	★★★★★
IMMUNITY	★★★★★
DIGESTION	★★★☆☆
SKIN	★★★★☆

219 | veggie cocktail

3 sticks celery
3 tomatoes
2 carrots
$\frac{1}{2}$ lemon

A sweet, pale orange vegetable juice – you could add
some parsley too if you want that green, cleansing taste.

NUTRIENTS

Beta-carotene, biotin, folic acid,
vitamin C; calcium, magnesium,
manganese, phosphorus, potassium,
sodium, sulphur

ENERGY	★★★★☆
DETOX	★★★☆☆
IMMUNITY	★★★★★
DIGESTION	★☆☆☆☆
SKIN	★★★★☆

220 | celery blood cleanser

3 sticks celery
1 apple
1 beet (beetroot)
1 teaspoon spirulina

You can hardly believe this is so good for you, it has such a fantastic
taste. Put in a little less beet if you're not a hardened fan. Shake the
spirulina with some of the juice in a jar before mixing in with the rest.

NUTRIENTS

Beta-carotene, folic acid, vitamins B1, B3,
B5, B6 and C; calcium, iron, magnesium,
manganese, phosphorus, potassium, sodium,
sulphur; protein, essential fatty acids

ENERGY	★★★☆☆
DETOX	★★★★★
IMMUNITY	★★★☆☆
DIGESTION	★★★★☆
SKIN	★★★★☆

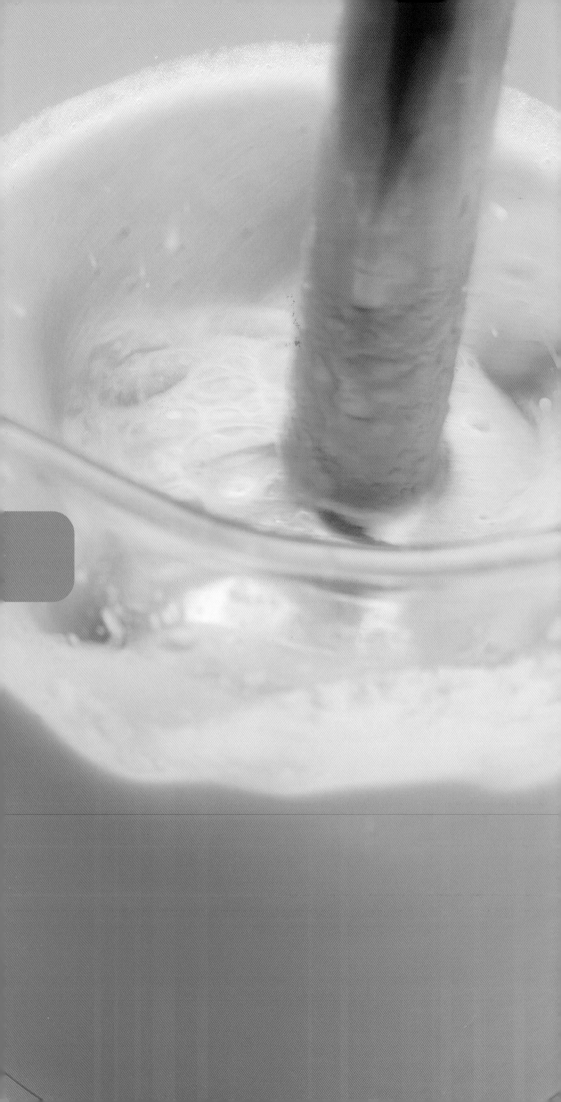

making
smoothies

chapter 3

Making a smoothie couldn't be easier – just prepare your ingredients (see pp.14–24), throw them into a blender and press "on".

In this chapter, fruity smoothies are thick drinks made from fresh fruits blended together with a little added fruit juice; and creamy smoothies are a richer, creamier drink because they contain yogurt. All of the creamy smoothie recipes list yogurt, but you can use milk or soy (soya) milk instead if you prefer a runnier drink. Either way, a creamy smoothie provides a rich source of protein.

Each recipe suggests which juice to add to help make your smoothie a drink, rather than a pudding, but feel free to experiment with different juices and different amounts according to your tastes and preferences. The recipes each make two generous portions, and provide a delicious, substantial drink, snack or even light meal for any time of the day.

top tips

Below are a few reminders and helpful hints, tips and suggestions to enable you to get the most from your smoothie making.

1   Choose fruit for a smoothie at its peak of ripeness for the best taste and most goodness in a glass.

2   When adding juice to your smoothie, use fresh, home-made juice in preference to commercially produced juices (which often contain artificial sweeteners and other additives).

3   When adding juice to your smoothie, you don't have to stick rigidly to the one listed in the ingredients – try using whichever juice you have available rather than go without.

4   Add more or less juice to your smoothie, according to your own tastes and preferences to make a thicker or thinner drink.

5   For creamy smoothies, the recipes suggest using yogurt. For thinner, runnier drinks, use milk or a milk alternative made from soy (soya), rice or nuts.

6   Use soy (soya) yogurt or soy (soya) milk as a non-dairy alternative when making creamy smoothies.

7   For a more refreshing smoothie, blend a few crushed cubes of ice in with the other ingredients.

8   Any smoothie can be frozen to be eaten as a delicious popsicle (ice-lolly). Either use special popsicle moulds or ice cube trays.

9   Try adding some of the extra ingredients listed on pp.24–5 to give your smoothie an even greater healthy boost.

10 Even if you don't have all the fruits needed for a particular recipe, or the exact amounts, give it a try anyway and have some fun creating your own blends.

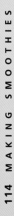

221 | pink banana

2 bananas
8 medium strawberries
10 tablespoons (150 ml) apple juice

This one is a summer favourite – best to use organic, fresh strawberries.

NUTRIENTS

Beta-carotene, biotin, folic acid,
vitamins B1, B3, B6 and C; calcium,
magnesium, phosphorus, potassium,
sulphur

ENERGY	★★★★★
DETOX	★☆☆☆☆
IMMUNITY	★★★☆☆
DIGESTION	★☆☆☆☆
SKIN	★★★☆☆

222 | green banana smoothie

1 banana
½ pineapple
8 tablespoons (120 ml) pineapple juice
2 tablespoons (30 ml) coconut milk
1 heaped teaspoon spirulina

The spirulina turns this delicious, pastel yellow drink into a green delight.

NUTRIENTS

Beta-carotene, folic acid, vitamins B1, B3, B6
and C; calcium, iron, magnesium, manganese,
phosphorus, potassium, sodium, sulphur;
protein, essential fatty acids

ENERGY	★★★★★
DETOX	★★★☆☆
IMMUNITY	★★★☆☆
DIGESTION	★★★★☆
SKIN	★★★☆☆

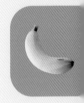

223 | green banana too

2 bananas
2 kiwi fruits
1 handful red seedless grapes
10 tablespoons (150 ml) apple juice

This one goes a pretty, green colour because of the delicious, tangy,
vitamin C-rich kiwi fruit.

NUTRIENTS

Beta-carotene, folic acid, vitamins B1, B3, B6,
C and E; calcium, magnesium, manganese,
phosphorus, potassium, sodium, sulphur

ENERGY	★★★★★
DETOX	★★★★☆
IMMUNITY	★★★★☆
DIGESTION	★★★☆☆
SKIN	★★★★☆

224 | banana sharp

2 bananas
1 pink grapefruit
8 tablespoons (120 ml) orange juice
juice of a lime

A great contrast between the tangy citrus and sweet banana.

NUTRIENTS

Beta-carotene, folic acid, vitamins B1, B3,
B6 and C; calcium, magnesium, phosphorus,
potassium, sodium, sulphur

ENERGY	★★★★★
DETOX	★☆☆☆☆
IMMUNITY	★★★☆☆
DIGESTION	★☆☆☆☆
SKIN	★★★☆☆

225 | pink lady

2 bananas
2 handfuls raspberries
10 tablespoons (150 ml) cranberry juice

This one is certainly heaven-sent and gives a great energy boost too.

NUTRIENTS

Beta-carotene, biotin, folic acid,
vitamins B1, B3, B6 and C; calcium, iron,
magnesium, manganese, phosphorus,
potassium, sodium, sulphur

ENERGY	★★★★★
DETOX	★☆☆☆☆
IMMUNITY	★★★☆☆
DIGESTION	★★☆☆☆
SKIN	★★★☆☆

226 | pure passion

3 bananas
4 passion fruits
10 tablespoons (150 ml) guava juice

Surely one of the most exquisite combinations of fruit ever.

NUTRIENTS

Beta-carotene, folic acid, vitamins B1,
B3, B6 and C; calcium, iron, magnesium,
phosphorus, potassium, sodium, sulphur

ENERGY	★★★★★
DETOX	★☆☆☆☆
IMMUNITY	★★★☆☆
DIGESTION	★☆☆☆☆
SKIN	★★★☆☆

227 | black banana

2 bananas
2 heaped tablespoons blackcurrants
10 tablespoons (150 ml) apple juice (or the juice from
    the blackcurrants, if they come from a can)

A wonderful contrast between the sweet banana and the
tangy blackcurrants. Use blackcurrants canned in natural
juice if you don't have fresh ones – a good standby to
keep in the cupboard in winter.

NUTRIENTS

Beta-carotene, biotin, vitamins B1,
B3, B6, C and E; calcium, iron,
magnesium, phosphorus,
potassium, sodium, sulphur

ENERGY ★★★★★
DETOX ★☆☆☆☆
IMMUNITY ★★★☆☆
DIGESTION ★☆☆☆☆
SKIN ★★★☆☆

228 | banana nectar

2 bananas
4 apricots
10 tablespoons (150 ml) apricot or apple juice

Nothing to do with nectarines – I always think the pulp or juice of apricots
conjures up the word nectar more than most fruits.

NUTRIENTS

Beta-carotene, folic acid, vitamins B1, B3, B6
and C; calcium, magnesium, phosphorus,
potassium, sulphur

ENERGY ★★★★★
DETOX ★☆☆☆☆
IMMUNITY ★★★☆☆
DIGESTION ★★☆☆☆
SKIN ★★★☆☆

229 | easy morning mash

2 bananas
1 pear
1 orange
8 tablespoons (120 ml) apple juice

Just reach into the fruit bowl and whiz it all up. Easy.

NUTRIENTS

Beta-carotene, folic acid, vitamins B1,
B3, B6 and C; calcium, magnesium,
phosphorus, potassium, sulphur

ENERGY	★★★★★
DETOX	★☆☆☆☆
IMMUNITY	★★★☆☆
DIGESTION	★★☆☆☆
SKIN	★★☆☆☆

230 | banana pie

2 bananas
1 apple
1 handful blackberries (or blackcurrants)
10 tablespoons (150 ml) apple juice

Well, not literally, but I always think of the apple and blackberry
pie combination when the two are blended and they cut deliciously
through the dense flavour of the banana.

NUTRIENTS

Beta-carotene, folic acid, vitamins B1,
B3, B5, B6, C and E; calcium, iron,
magnesium, phosphorus, potassium,
sodium, sulphur

ENERGY	★★★★★
DETOX	★☆☆☆☆
IMMUNITY	★★★☆☆
DIGESTION	★★☆☆☆
SKIN	★★☆☆☆

231 | tropical treat

1 banana
½ pineapple
½ papaya
8 tablespoons (120 ml) guava juice

Fancy being transported to a fresh fruit salad on a beach in Thailand?

NUTRIENTS

Beta-carotene, folic acid, vitamin B3,
vitamin C; calcium, magnesium, manganese,
phosphorus, potassium, sodium, sulphur

ENERGY	★★★★★
DETOX	★☆☆☆☆
IMMUNITY	★★★☆☆
DIGESTION	★★★★☆
SKIN	★★★☆☆

232 | peaches 'n' dream

2 bananas
2 peaches
2 tangerines
8 tablespoons (120 ml) orange juice

Juicy, ripe peaches (or nectarines) make this one a dream combination.

NUTRIENTS

Beta-carotene, folic acid, vitamins B1,
B3, B6 and C; calcium, magnesium,
phosphorus, potassium, sodium, sulphur

ENERGY	★★★★★
DETOX	★☆☆☆☆
IMMUNITY	★★★☆☆
DIGESTION	★★☆☆☆
SKIN	★★☆☆☆

233 | mellow bite

2 bananas
½ melon
8 tablespoons (120 ml) apple juice
juice of a lime

The contrasting mild melon and sharp lime make quite an impact on
your tastebuds but are mellowed by the banana.

NUTRIENTS

Beta-carotene, folic acid, vitamins B1,
B3, B6 and C; calcium, iron, magnesium,
phosphorus, potassium, sodium, sulphur

ENERGY	★★★★★
DETOX	★☆☆☆☆
IMMUNITY	★★★☆☆
DIGESTION	★☆☆☆☆
SKIN	★★ ☆☆☆

234 | coconutty 'nana

2 bananas
½ pineapple
2 tablespoons (30 ml) coconut milk
8 tablespoons (120 ml) pineapple juice

If you're a fan of coconut, you'll love this one and the
way it transports you to a warm, palm-fringed beach.

NUTRIENTS

Beta-carotene, folic acid, vitamins B1,
B3, B6, C and E; calcium, magnesium,
manganese, phosphorus, potassium,
sodium, sulphur

ENERGY	★★★★★
DETOX	★☆☆☆☆
IMMUNITY	★★★☆☆
DIGESTION	★★★★☆
SKIN	★★☆☆☆

235 | regular banana

2 bananas
10 prunes (soaked and pitted)
½ teaspoon vanilla essence
10 tablespoons (150 ml) apple juice

You'd barely believe this was so good for keeping your guts
going, it tastes so delicious. Use particularly ripe bananas.

NUTRIENTS

Beta-carotene, folic acid, vitamins B1,
B3, B6 and C; calcium, magnesium,
phosphorus, potassium, sulphur

ENERGY	★★★★☆
DETOX	★☆☆☆☆
IMMUNITY	★★★☆☆
DIGESTION	★★★☆☆
SKIN	★★☆☆☆

236 | eve's delight

2 mangoes
2 apples
8 tablespoons (120 ml) apple juice

If she'd had anything to blend it with in Eden, surely it would have
been a juicy, ripe mango. This is one of my all-time favourite smoothies.

NUTRIENTS

Beta-carotene, folic acid, vitamin C,
vitamin E; calcium, iron, magnesium,
phosphorus, potassium, sodium,
sulphur

ENERGY	★★★★★
DETOX	★☆☆☆☆
IMMUNITY	★★★★☆
DIGESTION	★★★★☆
SKIN	★★☆☆☆

237 | mango crush

2 mangoes
2 oranges
juice of a lime
8 tablespoons (120 ml) apple juice

One pure orange colour, two different tastes, one
result – a fabulous smoothie where the creamy, sweet
mango contrasts well with the tangy orange.

NUTRIENTS

Beta-carotene, folic acid, vitamin C,
vitamin E; calcium, iron, magnesium,
phosphorus, potassium, sodium, sulphur

ENERGY	★★★★★
DETOX	★☆☆☆☆
IMMUNITY	★★★★★
DIGESTION	★☆☆☆☆
SKIN	★★★☆☆

238 | simple tropical

2 mangoes
1 banana
10 tablespoons (150 ml) orange juice

Dense and rich, this is a high energy blend. You can use pineapple
juice as an alternative to the orange for an extra tropical touch.

NUTRIENTS

Beta-carotene, folic acid, vitamins B1, B3,
B6, C and E; calcium, iron, magnesium,
phosphorus, potassium, sodium,
sulphur

ENERGY	★★★★★
DETOX	★☆☆☆☆
IMMUNITY	★★★☆☆
DIGESTION	★★☆☆☆
SKIN	★★★☆☆

239 | mango passion

2 mangoes
½ pineapple
2 passion fruits
8 tablespoons (120 ml) pineapple juice

I love any blend with passion fruit, but with pineapple and mango, mmm...

NUTRIENTS

Beta-carotene, folic acid, vitamins B3,
C and E; calcium, iron, magnesium,
manganese, phosphorus, potassium,
sodium, sulphur

ENERGY	★★★★★
DETOX	★☆☆☆☆
IMMUNITY	★★★★☆
DIGESTION	★★★★☆
SKIN	★★★☆☆

240 | manilla

2 mangoes
4 tangerines
½ teaspoon vanilla essence
8 tablespoons (120 ml) orange juice

Somehow the vanilla makes this taste even sweeter.

NUTRIENTS

Beta-carotene, folic acid, vitamin C,
vitamin E; calcium, iron, magnesium,
phosphorus, potassium, sodium,
sulphur

ENERGY	★★★★★
DETOX	★☆☆☆☆
IMMUNITY	★★★★★
DIGESTION	★☆☆☆☆
SKIN	★★★☆☆

241 | mango zingo

2 mangoes
1 grapefruit
$\frac{1}{4}$ inch (0.5 cm) grated ginger root
8 tablespoons (120 ml) apple juice

The slightly bitter grapefruit and spicy ginger blend beautifully with sweet, creamy mango to create this energy- and immunity-boosting drink.

NUTRIENTS

Beta-carotene, folic acid, vitamin C, vitamin E; calcium, iron, magnesium, phosphorus, potassium, sodium, sulphur

ENERGY	★★★★★
DETOX	★☆☆☆☆
IMMUNITY	★★★★★
DIGESTION	★★☆☆☆
SKIN	★★★☆☆

242 | summer mango special

2 mangoes
2 handfuls raspberries
juice of half a lemon
8 tablespoons (120 ml) apple juice

Just as those fantastic Indian mangoes are at the tail end of their season, the raspberries come in – catch this divine combination if you can, otherwise use any good mango.

NUTRIENTS

Beta-carotene, biotin, folic acid, vitamin C, vitamin E; calcium, iron, magnesium, manganese, phosphorus, potassium, sodium, sulphur

ENERGY	★★★★★
DETOX	★★☆☆☆
IMMUNITY	★★★☆☆
DIGESTION	★★☆☆☆
SKIN	★★☆☆☆

243 | tropical deluxe

2 mangoes
2 bananas
juice of a lime
8 tablespoons (120 ml) guava juice

There have to be very few, if any, smoothies that go down this well.

NUTRIENTS

Beta-carotene, folic acid, vitamins B1, B3, B6, C and E; calcium, iron, magnesium, phosphorus, potassium, sodium, sulphur

ENERGY	★★★★★
DETOX	★☆☆☆☆
IMMUNITY	★★★★☆
DIGESTION	★★☆☆☆
SKIN	★★★☆☆

244 | nectargo

2 mangoes
2 nectarines
1 orange
8 tablespoons (120 ml) orange juice

A triple-orange whammy with a taste to match. This is also an
excellent booster blend for the body's defences.

NUTRIENTS

Beta-carotene, folic acid, vitamin C,
vitamin E; calcium, iron, magnesium,
phosphorus, potassium, sodium,
sulphur

ENERGY	★★★★★
DETOX	★☆☆☆☆
IMMUNITY	★★★★★
DIGESTION	★☆☆☆☆
SKIN	★★★★☆

245 | mango blues

2 mangoes
2 handfuls blueberries
juice of a lime
8 tablespoons (120 ml) apple juice

Tropic and temperate fruits kicking
up a storm in frothy red.

NUTRIENTS

Beta-carotene, biotin, folic acid,
vitamins B1, B2, B6, C and E; calcium,
chromium, iron, magnesium, phosphorus,
potassium, sodium, sulphur

ENERGY	★★★★★
DETOX	★★☆☆☆
IMMUNITY	★★★★★
DIGESTION	★★☆☆☆
SKIN	★★★★☆

246 | pineapple classic

½ pineapple
2 bananas
2 passion fruits
8 tablespoons (120 ml) pineapple juice

An idyllic tropical combo.

NUTRIENTS

Beta-carotene, folic acid, vitamin B3,
vitamin C; calcium, iron, magnesium,
manganese, phosphorus, potassium,
sodium, sulphur

ENERGY	★★★★★
DETOX	★☆☆☆☆
IMMUNITY	★★★☆☆
DIGESTION	★★★☆☆
SKIN	★★★☆☆

247 | citrus pineapple

½ pineapple
2 oranges
juice of a lime
6 tablespoons (90 ml) orange juice

A blend of three tangy flavours to get your tastebuds singing.

NUTRIENTS

Beta-carotene, folic acid, vitamin C;
calcium, magnesium, manganese,
phosphorus, potassium, sodium

ENERGY	★★★★★
DETOX	★☆☆☆☆
IMMUNITY	★★★★☆
DIGESTION	★★☆☆☆
SKIN	★★☆☆☆

248 | pineapple zing

½ pineapple
1 grapefruit
¼ inch (0.5 cm) grated ginger root
8 tablespoons (120 ml) pineapple juice

If you don't use a sweet, pink grapefruit for this one, you'll be in
for a sharp surprise. You decide.

NUTRIENTS

Beta-carotene, folic acid, vitamin C;
calcium, magnesium, manganese,
phosphorus, potassium, sodium,
sulphur,

ENERGY	★★★★★
DETOX	★☆☆☆☆
IMMUNITY	★★★★☆
DIGESTION	★★★☆☆
SKIN	★★★☆☆

249 | summer refresher

$\frac{3}{4}$ pineapple
1 handful raspberries
5–6 fresh mint leaves
8 tablespoons (120 ml) pineapple juice

A tropic-temperate blend of fruits lifted even higher with the
refreshing mint.

NUTRIENTS

Beta-carotene, biotin, folic acid,
vitamin C; calcium, magnesium,
manganese, phosphorus, potassium,
sodium, sulphur

ENERGY	★★★★★
DETOX	★☆☆☆☆
IMMUNITY	★★★☆☆
DIGESTION	★★★☆☆
SKIN	★★★☆☆

250 | pastel perfect

$\frac{1}{2}$ pineapple
3 kiwi fruits
8 tablespoons (120 ml) pineapple juice

A delicious mix that can be sharp on the tongue if the fruits aren't nice
and ripe, so pick your moment well.

NUTRIENTS

Beta-carotene, folic acid, vitamin C;
calcium, magnesium, manganese,
phosphorus, potassium, sodium

ENERGY	★★★★★
DETOX	★★☆☆☆
IMMUNITY	★★★★☆
DIGESTION	★★★☆☆
SKIN	★★★☆☆

251 | malibu mix

1 pineapple
2 tablespoons (30 ml) coconut milk
$\frac{1}{2}$ teaspoon vanilla essence
juice of $\frac{1}{2}$ lemon
5 tablespoons (75 ml) pineapple juice

Sit back and enjoy the sunshine. Well, perhaps the central heating … .
Either way, it's very good and will transport you to tropical climes.

NUTRIENTS

Beta-carotene, folic acid, vitamin C,
vitamin E; calcium, magnesium,
manganese, phosphorus, potassium,
sodium, sulphur

ENERGY	★★★★★
DETOX	★★☆☆☆
IMMUNITY	★★☆☆☆
DIGESTION	★★★☆☆
SKIN	★★☆☆☆

252 | pineberry

½ pineapple
1 handful cranberries
1 handful strawberries
8 tablespoons (120 ml) pineapple juice

The sharp taste of the cranberries is well balanced
by the sweetness of all the other ingredients.

NUTRIENTS

Beta-carotene, biotin, folic acid,
vitamin C; calcium, iron, magnesium,
manganese, phosphorus, potassium,
sodium, sulphur

ENERGY	★★★★★
DETOX	★★☆☆☆
IMMUNITY	★★★★☆
DIGESTION	★★☆☆☆
SKIN	★★★☆☆

253 | apple squared

½ pineapple
2 apples
8 tablespoons (120 ml) apple juice

I was surprised at how well this combination worked out! Use a
relatively sweet apple variety, such as Pink Lady or Empire, for
the perfect contrast.

NUTRIENTS

Beta-carotene, folic acid, vitamin C;
calcium, magnesium, manganese,
phosphorus, potassium, sodium,
sulphur

ENERGY	★★★★★
DETOX	★☆☆☆☆
IMMUNITY	★★★☆☆
DIGESTION	★★★★☆
SKIN	★★★☆☆

254 | papaya pure

2 papayas
juice of a lime
8 tablespoons (120 ml) apple juice

This, the first of three Thai-inspired recipes, is pure Thailand in a glass –
whenever you buy a slice of fresh papaya from a street stall in this tropical
country, it is always served with a wedge of lime.

NUTRIENTS

Beta-carotene, folic acid, vitamin C;
calcium, magnesium, phosphorus,
potassium, sodium, sulphur

ENERGY	★★★★★
DETOX	★★★★☆
IMMUNITY	★★★★☆
DIGESTION	★★★★☆
SKIN	★★★★☆

255 | papaya salad

1 papaya
$\frac{1}{4}$ pineapple
1 slice watermelon
1 banana
8 tablespoons (120 ml) pineapple juice

This classic combo served to tropical-fruit-hungry foreigners for breakfast
in Thailand is a delicious smoothie in any corner of the globe.

NUTRIENTS

Beta-carotene, folic acid, vitamins B1,
B3, B5, B6 and C; calcium, magnesium,
manganese, phosphorus, potassium,
sodium, sulphur

ENERGY	★★★★★
DETOX	★★★☆☆
IMMUNITY	★★★★☆
DIGESTION	★★★★☆
SKIN	★★★★☆

256 | identity crisis

1 papaya
3 tangerines
8 tablespoons (120 ml) orange juice

In Thailand, "oranges" are usually green and taste like tangerines.
Whatever ... this is a wonderfully refreshing blend.

NUTRIENTS

Beta-carotene, folic acid, vitamin C;
calcium, magnesium, phosphorus,
potassium, sodium

ENERGY	★★★★★
DETOX	★☆☆☆☆
IMMUNITY	★★★★★
DIGESTION	★★☆☆☆
SKIN	★★★☆☆

257 | heaven scent

1 papaya
1 grapefruit
1 handful raspberries
juice of a lime
8 tablespoons (120 ml) grapefruit juice

Quite a magnificent combination of tastes.

NUTRIENTS

Beta-carotene, biotin, folic acid,
vitamin C; calcium, magnesium,
manganese, phosphorus, potassium,
sodium, sulphur

ENERGY	★★★★★
DETOX	★☆☆☆☆
IMMUNITY	★★★★★
DIGESTION	★☆☆☆☆
SKIN	★★★★☆

258 | globe trotter

1 papaya
2 kiwi fruits
1 pear
8 tablespoons (120 ml) apple juice

This one is certainly a sign of the times – fruit from around the world
in one big taste.

NUTRIENTS

Beta-carotene, folic acid, vitamin C;
calcium, magnesium, phosphorus,
potassium, sodium, sulphur

ENERGY	★★★★★
DETOX	★☆☆☆☆
IMMUNITY	★★★★☆
DIGESTION	★★★☆☆
SKIN	★★★★☆

259 | supreme strawberry

2 handfuls strawberries
2 oranges
8 tablespoons (120 ml) guava juice

The most popular berry just got even better.

NUTRIENTS

Beta-carotene, folic acid, biotin,
vitamin B3, vitamin C; calcium,
magnesium, phosphorus, potassium,
sodium, sulphur

ENERGY	★★★★★
DETOX	★☆☆☆☆
IMMUNITY	★★★★★
DIGESTION	☆☆☆☆☆
SKIN	★★★★☆

260 | strawblend classic

2 handfuls strawberries
1 banana
$\frac{1}{4}$ pineapple
8 tablespoons (120 ml) pineapple juice

Classic favourites, strawberries and banana, with a touch
of tang from the tropics create this fabulous staple blend.

NUTRIENTS

Beta-carotene, biotin, folic acid,
vitamins B1, B3, B6 and C; calcium,
magnesium, manganese, phosphorus,
potassium, sodium, sulphur

ENERGY	★★★★★
DETOX	★☆☆☆☆
IMMUNITY	★★★★☆
DIGESTION	★★☆☆☆
SKIN	★★★★☆

261 | peachy strawbs

2 handfuls strawberries
3 peaches (or nectarines)
juice of one lime
8 tablespoons (120 ml) orange juice

Summer delight in a glass, and laden with antioxidants for better
immunity and healthy skin.

NUTRIENTS

Beta-carotene, biotin, folic acid,
vitamin B3, vitamin C; calcium,
magnesium, phosphorus, potassium,
sodium, sulphur

ENERGY	★★★★★
DETOX	★★☆☆☆
IMMUNITY	★★★★★
DIGESTION	☆☆☆☆☆
SKIN	★★★★★

262 | pink berry crush

2 handfuls raspberries
2 handfuls strawberries
1 orange
3 or 4 fresh mint leaves
8 tablespoons (120 ml) orange juice

An easy summer favourite with a hint of mint.

NUTRIENTS

Beta-carotene, biotin, folic acid,
vitamin C; calcium, magnesium,
manganese, phosphorus, potassium,
sodium, sulphur

ENERGY	★★★★★
DETOX	★★☆☆☆
IMMUNITY	★★★★★
DIGESTION	★☆☆☆☆
SKIN	★★★★★

263 | citrus strawbs

2 handfuls strawberries
1 pink grapefruit
2 oranges
6 tablespoons (90 ml) orange juice

Another strawberry blend that'll have you coming back for more and more.

NUTRIENTS

Beta-carotene, biotin, folic acid,
vitamin C; calcium, magnesium,
phosphorus, potassium, sulphur

ENERGY	★★★★★
DETOX	★★☆☆☆
IMMUNITY	★★★★☆
DIGESTION	☆☆☆☆☆
SKIN	★★★☆☆

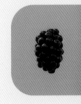

264 | berry bonanza II

1 handful raspberries
1 handful strawberries
1 handful blueberries
1 handful blackberries
8 tablespoons (120 ml) apple juice

Just use every type of berry they've got at the shop to create this high-energy, immunity-boosting combo.

NUTRIENTS

Beta-carotene, biotin, folic acid,
vitamins B1, B2, B6, C and E; calcium,
chromium, iron, magnesium, manganese,
phosphorus, potassium, sodium, sulphur

ENERGY	★★★★★
DETOX	★★☆☆☆
IMMUNITY	★★★★★
DIGESTION	★☆☆☆☆
SKIN	★★★★☆

265 | blue healer

1 handful blueberries
1 handful blackberries
1 handful blackcurrants
1 banana
10 tablespoons (150 ml) apple juice

Named after a boisterous breed of dog in Australia, this is a rich mix.

NUTRIENTS

Beta-carotene, biotin, folic acid,
vitamins B1, B2, B3, B5, B6, C and E;
calcium, chromium, iron, magnesium,
manganese, phosphorus, potassium,
sodium, sulphur

ENERGY	★★★★★
DETOX	★☆☆☆☆
IMMUNITY	★★★★★
DIGESTION	★★☆☆☆
SKIN	★★★★☆

266 | apple and black

2 handfuls blackberries
1 handful blackcurrants
2 apples
10 tablespoons (150 ml) apple juice

It's that favourite pie or crumble combination again, without the topping.

NUTRIENTS

Beta-carotene, biotin, folic acid,
vitamins B5, C and E; calcium, iron,
magnesium, phosphorus, potassium,
sodium, sulphur

ENERGY	★★★★★
DETOX	★☆☆☆☆
IMMUNITY	★★★★☆
DIGESTION	★★☆☆☆
SKIN	★★★★★

267 | cranapple crush

2 handfuls raspberries
1 handful cranberries
2 apples
10 tablespoons (150 ml) apple juice

Contrasting berries and sweet apples make a delicious drink.

NUTRIENTS

Beta-carotene, biotin, folic acid, vitamin C;
calcium, iron, magnesium, manganese,
phosphorus, potassium, sodium, sulphur

ENERGY	★★★★★
DETOX	★★☆☆☆
IMMUNITY	★★★★★
DIGESTION	☆☆☆☆☆
SKIN	★★★☆☆

268 | panana

3 peaches (or nectarines)
2 bananas
10 tablespoons (150 ml) apple juice

Creamy and sweet – a complete treat.

NUTRIENTS

Beta-carotene, folic acid, vitamins B1, B3,
B6 and C; calcium, magnesium, phosphorus,
potassium, sodium, sulphur

ENERGY	★★★★★
DETOX	★☆☆☆☆
IMMUNITY	★★★★☆
DIGESTION	★★★☆☆
SKIN	★★★★☆

269 | peach melba

3 peaches (or nectarines)
1 banana
1 handful raspberries
10 tablespoons (150 ml) apple juice

An exquisite combination bursting with energy and taste.

NUTRIENTS

Beta-carotene, biotin, folic acid,
vitamins B1, B3, B6 and C; calcium,
magnesium, manganese, phosphorus,
potassium, sodium, sulphur

ENERGY	★★★★★
DETOX	★☆☆☆☆
IMMUNITY	★★★★☆
DIGESTION	★★☆☆☆
SKIN	★★★☆☆

270 | summer sunset

3 peaches (or nectarines)
2 handfuls strawberries
10 tablespoons (150 ml) guava juice

You won't be able to stop drinking this one – heaven on a summer's day.

NUTRIENTS

Beta-carotene, biotin, folic acid,
vitamin B3, vitamin C; calcium,
magnesium, phosphorus, potassium,
sodium, sulphur

ENERGY	★★★★★
DETOX	★☆☆☆☆
IMMUNITY	★★★★★
DIGESTION	☆☆☆☆☆
SKIN	★★★★★

271 | creamy orange dream

3 peaches (or nectarines)
1 mango
1 orange
8 tablespoons (120 ml) orange juice

Three different orange-coloured fruit, with wonderfully
contrasting tastes and textures.

NUTRIENTS

Beta-carotene, folic acid, vitamin B3,
vitamin C; calcium, iron, magnesium,
phosphorus, potassium, sodium, sulphur

ENERGY ★★★★★
DETOX ★☆☆☆☆
IMMUNITY ★★★★★
DIGESTION ★☆☆☆☆
SKIN ★★★★★

272 | orangicot

5 apricots
2 oranges
8 tablespoons (120 ml) orange juice

Tangy and refreshing, with creamy apricots to take the edge
off the sharper oranges. Brimming with antioxidants.

NUTRIENTS

Beta-carotene, folic acid,
vitamins B1, B3, B5 and C; calcium,
magnesium, phosphorus, potassium,
sulphur

ENERGY ★★★★★
DETOX ★☆☆☆☆
IMMUNITY ★★★★★
DIGESTION ★☆☆☆☆
SKIN ★★★★★

273 | apricot zinger

5 apricots
2 pears
$\frac{1}{4}$ inch (0.5 cm) grated ginger root
10 tablespoons (150 ml) apple juice

A surprising combination which blends beautifully thanks to the hot ginger contrasting with the rich, sweeter apricots.

NUTRIENTS

Beta-carotene, folic acid, vitamins B3, B5 and C; calcium, magnesium, phosphorus, potassium, sulphur

ENERGY	★★★★★
DETOX	★☆☆☆☆
IMMUNITY	★★★★★
DIGESTION	★★★☆☆
SKIN	★★★★★

274 | sweet 'n' smooth

10 apricots
juice of half a lime
10 tablespoons (150 ml) prune juice

The sweetness of these two combined is fantastic, not to mention good for keeping your guts going.

NUTRIENTS

Beta-carotene, folic acid, vitamins B3, B5 and C; calcium, magnesium, phosphorus, potassium, sulphur

ENERGY	★★★★★
DETOX	★☆☆☆☆
IMMUNITY	★★★★★
DIGESTION	★★★★★
SKIN	★★★★★

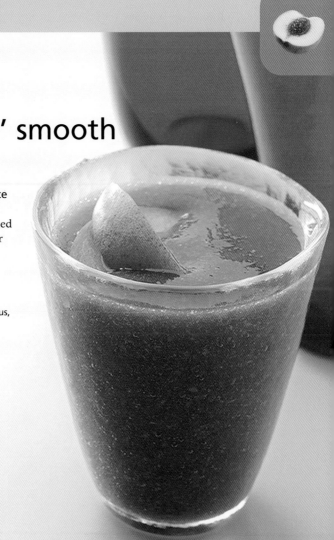

275 | pure watermelon

1 small watermelon (or 4 thick slices)

The fruit, the whole fruit and nothing but the fruit. The ground-up
seeds add a nutty, not to mention nutritious, touch.

NUTRIENTS

Beta-carotene, folic acid, vitamin B5,
vitamin C; calcium, magnesium,
phosphorus, potassium, sodium

ENERGY	★★★★★
DETOX	★★★★☆
IMMUNITY	★★★★★
DIGESTION	★★☆☆☆
SKIN	★★★★★

276 | watermelon crush

$\frac{1}{2}$ small watermelon (or 2 thick slices)
2 handfuls raspberries

A tastebud sensation, and as for the colour…

NUTRIENTS

Beta-carotene, biotin, folic acid,
vitamin B5, vitamin C; calcium,
magnesium, manganese, phosphorus,
potassium, sodium, sulphur

ENERGY	★★★★★
DETOX	★★☆☆☆
IMMUNITY	★★★★★
DIGESTION	★☆☆☆☆
SKIN	★★★★★

277 | creamy cooler

$\frac{1}{2}$ small watermelon (or 2 thick slices)
1 mango

Bubbling, refreshing and sweet – you can only swallow this down in huge,
noisy, full-of-goodness gulps.

NUTRIENTS

Beta-carotene, folic acid, vitamins B5,
C and E; calcium, iron, magnesium,
phosphorus, potassium, sodium, sulphur

ENERGY	★★★★★
DETOX	★☆☆☆☆
IMMUNITY	★★★★☆
DIGESTION	★★☆☆☆
SKIN	★★★★☆

278 | melon zinger

½ melon
½ pineapple
¼ inch (0.5 cm) grated ginger root

There's something about this blend that makes the result infinitely greater than the sum of its already fantastic parts.

NUTRIENTS

Beta-carotene, folic acid, vitamin C; calcium, magnesium, manganese, phosphorus, potassium, sodium, sulphur

ENERGY	★★★★★
DETOX	★★☆☆☆
IMMUNITY	★★★★☆
DIGESTION	★★★★☆
SKIN	★★★★☆

279 | green sensation

½ melon
2 kiwi fruits
1 pear
juice of half a lime
4 tablespoons (60 ml) apple juice

Three refreshing fruits blended with juice to make a kicking smoothie.

NUTRIENTS

Beta-carotene, folic acid, vitamin C; calcium, magnesium, phosphorus, potassium, sodium, sulphur

ENERGY	★★★★★
DETOX	★★★☆☆
IMMUNITY	★★★★☆
DIGESTION	★★☆☆☆
SKIN	★★★★☆

280 | melon sour

1 melon
juice of 2 limes
1 stick celery (with string well removed)
5–6 fresh mint leaves
4 tablespoons (60 ml) apple juice

A great, refreshing cocktail to awaken those sour tastebuds.

NUTRIENTS

Beta-carotene, folic acid, vitamin C; calcium, magnesium, phosphorus, potassium, sodium, sulphur

ENERGY	★★★★★
DETOX	★★☆☆☆
IMMUNITY	★★★★☆
DIGESTION	☆☆☆☆☆
SKIN	★★★☆☆

281 | creamy pure banana

2 bananas
5 tablespoons (75 ml) natural yogurt
10 tablespoons (150 ml) pineapple juice

Probably the original smoothie – bananas just ask to be made up into
a thick, creamy blend like this.

NUTRIENTS

Beta-carotene, folic acid, vitamins B1,
B3, B6 and C; calcium, magnesium,
manganese, phosphorus, potassium,
sulphur, zinc; protein

ENERGY	★★★★☆
DETOX	☆☆☆☆☆
IMMUNITY	★★☆☆☆
DIGESTION	★★★★☆
SKIN	★★★☆☆

282 | creamy bananacot

2 bananas
4 apricots
5 tablespoons (75 ml) natural yogurt
10 tablespoons (150 ml) apricot or apple juice

When an apricot is ripe, it is food from the heavens.
You can make this in winter with apricots canned in juice.

NUTRIENTS

Beta-carotene, folic acid, vitamins B1,
B3, B5, B6 and C; calcium, magnesium,
phosphorus, potassium, sulphur,
zinc; protein

ENERGY	★★★★☆
DETOX	☆☆☆☆☆
IMMUNITY	★★★☆☆
DIGESTION	★★★★☆
SKIN	★★★☆☆

283 | creamy black banana

1 banana
2 heaped tablespoons blackcurrants
5 tablespoons (75 ml) natural yogurt
10 tablespoons (150 ml) apple juice (or the juice from the
blackcurrants, if they come from a can)

This is my all-time favourite combination – the rich banana and tangy blackcurrants.
You can even make it throughout the winter using blackcurrants canned in natural
juice. Try crunching on the blackcurrant seeds as they are full of healthy oils.

NUTRIENTS

Beta-carotene, biotin, vitamins B1, B3, B5,
B6, C and E; calcium, magnesium, phosphorus,
potassium, sodium, sulphur, zinc; protein

ENERGY	★★★★☆
DETOX	☆☆☆☆☆
IMMUNITY	★★★★☆
DIGESTION	★★★☆☆
SKIN	★★★★☆

284 | creamy pink banana

1 banana
2 handfuls strawberries
5 tablespoons (75 ml) natural yogurt
8 tablespoons (120 ml) apple juice

Another favourite combination of mine – best in the summer with juicy, fresh,
flavoursome, organic strawberries.

NUTRIENTS

Beta-carotene, biotin, folic acid,
vitamins B1, B3, B6 and C; calcium,
magnesium, phosphorus, potassium,
sulphur, zinc; protein

ENERGY	★★★★☆
DETOX	☆☆☆☆☆
IMMUNITY	★★★★☆
DIGESTION	★★★☆☆
SKIN	★★★★☆

285 | creamy green banana

1 banana
$\frac{1}{4}$ pineapple
1 heaped teaspoon spirulina
5 tablespoons (75 ml) natural yogurt
6 tablespoons (90 ml) pineapple juice

This isn't to say you should use green bananas, but you turn a pale yellow
smoothie into a pastel green by adding the spirulina.

NUTRIENTS

Beta-carotene, folic acid, vitamins B1,
B3, B5, B6 and C; calcium, iron, magnesium,
manganese, phosphorus, potassium, sodium,
sulphur, zinc; protein, essential fatty acids

ENERGY	★★★★☆
DETOX	★★★☆☆
IMMUNITY	★★★☆☆
DIGESTION	★★★★☆
SKIN	★★☆☆☆

286 | tropical tang

1 banana
½ mango
½ pineapple
4 tablespoons (50 ml) pineapple juice
5 tablespoons (75 ml) natural yogurt

This one reminds me of my first backpacking trip to an idyllic beach in Thailand when smoothies were only on the menu for a couple of hours a day – when the generator was turned on and the blender could be powered up.

NUTRIENTS

Beta-carotene, folic acid, vitamins B1, B3, B6, C and E; calcium, iron, magnesium, manganese, phosphorus, potassium, sodium, sulphur, zinc; protein

ENERGY	★★★★☆
DETOX	★☆☆☆☆
IMMUNITY	★★★★☆
DIGESTION	★★★★☆
SKIN	★★★☆☆

287 | vanilla banana

2 bananas
8 rehydrated prunes
3 drops vanilla essence
5 tablespoons (75 ml) natural yogurt
6 tablespoons (90 ml) pineapple juice

This turns out a tasty, very sweet smoothie. If you don't have any prunes to hand or don't like them, use dried apricots instead. Both are best left to soak overnight first.

NUTRIENTS

Beta-carotene, folic acid, vitamins B1, B3, B6 and C; calcium, magnesium, manganese, phosphorus, potassium, sodium, sulphur, zinc; protein

ENERGY	★★★★★
DETOX	★☆☆☆☆
IMMUNITY	★★★★☆
DIGESTION	★★★★☆
SKIN	★★★☆☆

288 | creamy passion

2 bananas
4 passion fruits
5 tablespoons (75 ml) natural yogurt
10 tablespoons (150 ml) guava juice

Surely one of the most exquisite combinations of fruit ever, bound up with creamy yogurt into a thick meal in itself.

NUTRIENTS

Beta-carotene, folic acid, vitamin B1, B3, B6 and C; calcium, iron, magnesium, phosphorus, potassium, sodium, sulphur; protein

ENERGY	★★★★☆
DETOX	☆☆☆☆☆
IMMUNITY	★★★☆☆
DIGESTION	★★★☆☆
SKIN	★★☆☆☆

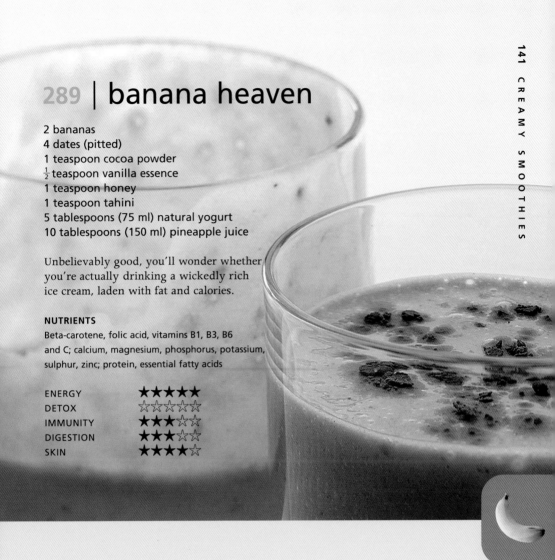

289 | banana heaven

2 bananas
4 dates (pitted)
1 teaspoon cocoa powder
½ teaspoon vanilla essence
1 teaspoon honey
1 teaspoon tahini
5 tablespoons (75 ml) natural yogurt
10 tablespoons (150 ml) pineapple juice

Unbelievably good, you'll wonder whether
you're actually drinking a wickedly rich
ice cream, laden with fat and calories.

NUTRIENTS

Beta-carotene, folic acid, vitamins B1, B3, B6
and C; calcium, magnesium, phosphorus, potassium,
sulphur, zinc; protein, essential fatty acids

ENERGY	★★★★★
DETOX	☆☆☆☆☆
IMMUNITY	★★★☆☆
DIGESTION	★★★☆☆
SKIN	★★★★☆

290 | peachy banana dream

2 bananas
2 peaches
2 tangerines
5 tablespoons (75 ml) natural yogurt
8 tablespoons (120 ml) orange juice

Juicy, ripe peaches (or nectarines) make this one a dream combination,
full of energy, with the creaminess offset by the citrus.

NUTRIENTS

Beta-carotene, folic acid, vitamins B1, B3,
B6 and C; calcium, magnesium, phosphorus,
potassium, sodium, sulphur; zinc, protein

ENERGY	★★★★☆
DETOX	★☆☆☆☆
IMMUNITY	★★★★☆
DIGESTION	★★★☆☆
SKIN	★★★☆☆

291 | creamy pure mango

2 mangoes
$\frac{1}{4}$ teaspoon ground cardamom
5 tablespoons (75 ml) natural yogurt
6 tablespoons (90 ml) pineapple juice

Dense and rich, this is a high energy blend, with a hint of my favourite spice. Just leave it out if you don't like cardamom.

NUTRIENTS

Beta-carotene, folic acid, vitamin C, vitamin E; calcium, iron, magnesium, manganese, phosphorus, potassium, sodium, sulphur, zinc; protein

ENERGY	★★★★☆
DETOX	★★☆☆☆
IMMUNITY	★★★★☆
DIGESTION	★★★☆☆
SKIN	★★★☆☆

292 | magical mango

1 mango
1 banana
5 tablespoons (75 ml) natural yogurt
10 tablespoons (150 ml) orange juice

Creamy and sweet – free transport to the tropics included.

NUTRIENTS

Beta-carotene, folic acid, vitamins B1, B3, B6, C and E; calcium, iron, magnesium, phosphorus, potassium, sodium, sulphur, zinc; protein

ENERGY	★★★★☆
DETOX	☆☆☆☆☆
IMMUNITY	★★★☆☆
DIGESTION	★★★☆☆
SKIN	★★★☆☆

293 | mango mango

2 mangoes
5 tablespoons (75 ml) natural yogurt
6 tablespoons (90 ml) pineapple juice

One of the fruits that was just made to be blended with yogurt.

NUTRIENTS

Beta carotene, folic acid, vitamin C, vitamin E; calcium, iron, magnesium, manganese, phosphorus, potassium, sodium, sulphur, zinc; protein

ENERGY	★★★★☆
DETOXING	★☆☆☆☆
IMMUNITY	★★★★☆
DIGESTION	★★★★☆
SKIN	★★★☆☆

294 | pango mango

2 mangoes
2 peaches
$\frac{1}{2}$ teaspoon vanilla essence
5 tablespoons (75 ml) natural yogurt
8 tablespoons (120 ml) orange juice

Two fantastically fruity orange fruits taken to another realm
with the hint of vanilla, which seems to make it even sweeter.

NUTRIENTS

Beta-carotene, folic acid, vitamins B3,	ENERGY	★★★★☆
C and E; calcium, iron, magnesium,	DETOX	★☆☆☆☆
phosphorus, potassium, sodium,	IMMUNITY	★★★★☆
sulphur, zinc; protein	DIGESTION	★★★☆☆
	SKIN	★★★★☆

295 | pinky mango

2 mangoes
2 handfuls raspberries
juice of half a lemon
5 tablespoons (75 ml) natural yogurt
8 tablespoons (120 ml) apple juice

Who said East is East and West is West – the twain meet superbly here.

NUTRIENTS

Beta-carotene, biotin, folic acid, vitamin C,	ENERGY	★★★★☆
vitmain E; calcium, iron, magnesium,	DETOX	★☆☆☆☆
manganese, phosphorus, potassium,	IMMUNITY	★★★★☆
sodium, sulphur, zinc; protein	DIGESTION	★★★☆☆
	SKIN	★★★☆☆

296 | tropical mango medley

1 mango
$\frac{1}{2}$ pineapple
1 banana
1 passion fruit
5 tablespoons (75 ml) natural yogurt
6 tablespoons (90 ml) pineapple juice

A delicious, creamy drink redolent of breakfast on a palm-fringed beach.

NUTRIENTS

Beta carotene, folic acid, vitamins B1,	ENERGY	★★★★☆
B3, B6, C and E; calcium, iron,	DETOX	★☆☆☆☆
magnesium, manganese,phosphorus,	IMMUNITY	★★★★☆
potassium, sodium, sulphur, zinc; protein	DIGESTION	★★★★☆
	SKIN	★★★☆☆

297 | cocogo

2 mangoes
1 dessertspoon coconut milk
$\frac{1}{2}$ teaspoon vanilla essence
5 tablespoons (75 ml) natural yogurt
6 tablespoons (90 ml) pineapple juice

A sweet, creamy drink with the tropical taste of coconut. Another one to transport you to sunny climes.

NUTRIENTS

Beta-carotene, folic acid, vitamin C, vitamin E; calcium, iron, magnesium, phosphorus, potassium, sodium, sulphur, zinc; protein,

ENERGY	★★★★☆
DETOX	★☆☆☆☆
IMMUNITY	★★★★☆
DIGESTION	★★★☆☆
SKIN	★★★☆☆

298 | berry mango

1 mango
1 handful strawberries
$\frac{1}{4}$ pineapple
5 tablespoons (75 ml) natural yogurt
6 tablespoons (90 ml) pineapple juice

The tangy pineapple contrasts deliciously with the creamy mango and sweet strawberries.

NUTRIENTS

Beta-carotene, folic acid, vitamin C, vitamin E; calcium, iron, magnesium, manganese, phosphorus, potassium, sodium, sulphur, zinc; protein

ENERGY	★★★★☆
DETOX	★☆☆☆☆
IMMUNITY	★★★★☆
DIGESTION	★★★★☆
SKIN	★★★★☆

299 | flecked mango

2 mangoes
2 handfuls blueberries
5 tablespoons (75 ml) natural yogurt
8 tablespoons (120 ml) apple juice

I love the flecks of blue that the skins of the berries dot throughout
this drink, let alone the sublime taste they produce.

NUTRIENTS

Beta-carotene, biotin, folic acid,
vitamins B1, B2, B6, C and E;
calcium, chromium, iron, magnesium,
phosphorus, potassium, sodium,
sulphur, zinc; protein

ENERGY	★★★★☆
DETOX	★☆☆☆☆
IMMUNITY	★★★★☆
DIGESTION	★★★☆☆
SKIN	★★★☆☆

300 | passionate about mangoes

2 mangoes
2 tangerines
2 passion fruits
5 tablespoons (75 ml) natural yogurt
8 tablespoons (120 ml) pineapple juice

Just when you thought mangoes couldn't get any better, in jumps passion fruit,
and both are offset by the citrusy tangerines.

NUTRIENTS

Beta-carotene, folic acid, vitamins B3,
C and E; calcium, iron, magnesium,
phosphorus, potassium, sodium,
sulphur, zinc; protein

ENERGY	★★★★☆
DETOX	★☆☆☆☆
IMMUNITY	★★★★☆
DIGESTION	★★☆☆☆
SKIN	★★★☆☆

301 | pink melon

2 handfuls strawberries
$\frac{1}{2}$ melon
5 tablespoons (75 ml) natural yogurt
6 tablespoons (90 ml) apple juice

Even though I don't normally like melon
with yogurt, this blend is fantastic.

NUTRIENTS

Beta-carotene, biotin, folic acid,
vitamin C; calcium, magnesium,
phosphorus, potassium, sodium,
sulphur; protein

ENERGY	★★★★☆
DETOX	★☆☆☆☆
IMMUNITY	★★★★☆
DIGESTION	★★★☆☆
SKIN	★★★★☆

302 | pure pink thickie

2 handfuls strawberries
3 handfuls raspberries
5 tablespoons (75 ml) natural yogurt
6 tablespoons (90 ml) mineral water

Everybody's summer favourites in a thick, creamy drink. Berries lend
themselves perfectly to creamy smoothies.

NUTRIENTS

Beta-carotene, biotin, folic acid,
vitamin C; calcium, magnesium,
manganese, phosphorus, potassium,
sodium, sulphur; protein

ENERGY	★★★★☆
DETOX	★☆☆☆☆
IMMUNITY	★★★★☆
DIGESTION	★★☆☆☆
SKIN	★★★★☆

303 | creamy pink banana II

1 handful strawberries
1 handful raspberries
1 banana
5 tablespoons (75 ml) natural yogurt
6 tablespoons (90 ml) apple juice

Pink berry treats with another firm favourite.

NUTRIENTS

Beta-carotene, biotin, folic acid,
vitamins B1, B3, B6 and C; calcium,
magnesium, manganese, phosphorus,
potassium, sodium, sulphur; protein

ENERGY	★★★★☆
DETOX	★☆☆☆☆
IMMUNITY	★★★★☆
DIGESTION	★★★☆☆
SKIN	★★★☆☆

304 | tropical pinkie

1 handful strawberries
1 handful raspberries
$\frac{1}{2}$ pineapple
5 tablespoons (75 ml) natural yogurt
6 tablespoons (90 ml) pineapple juice

Pineapple crushes up fantastically with these succulent berries.

NUTRIENTS

Beta-carotene, biotin, folic acid,
vitamin C; calcium, magnesium,
manganese, phosphorus, potassium,
sodium, sulphur; protein

ENERGY	★★★★☆
DETOX	★☆☆☆☆
IMMUNITY	★★★★☆
DIGESTION	★★★☆☆
SKIN	★★★☆☆

305 | creamy berry tang

2 handfuls strawberries
2 handfuls raspberries
2 oranges
5 tablespoons (75 ml) natural yogurt
6 tablespoons (125 ml) guava juice

The guava juice really brings out the flavours in this one.

NUTRIENTS

Beta-carotene, biotin, folic acid,
vitamin B3, vitamin C; calcium,
magnesium, manganese, phosphorus,
potassium, sodium, sulphur; protein

ENERGY	★★★★☆
DETOX	★☆☆☆☆
IMMUNITY	★★★★☆
DIGESTION	★★☆☆☆
SKIN	★★★★☆

306 | purple rain

1 handful blueberries
1 handful blackberries
1 handful blackcurrants
5 tablespoons (75 ml) natural yogurt
6 tablespoons (90 ml) apple juice

Get them all in, any black or blue you can get your hands on, for a
powerful taste sensation, not to mention a glassful of goodness.

NUTRIENTS

Beta-carotene, biotin, folic acid,	ENERGY	★★★★☆
vitamins B1, B2, B5, B6, C and E;	DETOX	★☆☆☆☆
calcium, chromium, iron, magnesium,	IMMUNITY	★★★★☆
manganese, phosphorus, potassium,	DIGESTION	★★★☆☆
sodium, sulphur, zinc; protein	SKIN	★★★★☆

307 | mighty berry

4 handfuls blueberries, blackberries, blackcurrants,
  strawberries, raspberries
5 tablespoons (75 ml) natural yogurt
6 tablespoons (90 ml) cranberry juice

Purple Rain plus the red ones too – a serious berry bonanza in a creamy base.

NUTRIENTS

Beta-carotene, biotin, folic acid,	ENERGY	★★★★☆
vitamins B1, B2, B5, B6, C and E;	DETOX	★★☆☆☆
calcium, chromium, iron, magnesium,	IMMUNITY	★★★★☆
manganese, phosphorus, potassium,	DIGESTION	★★★☆☆
sodium, sulphur, zinc; protein	SKIN	★★★★☆

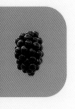

308 | purple 'nana

3 handfuls blueberries, blackberries, blackcurrants
1 banana
5 tablespoons (75 ml) natural yogurt
6 tablespoons (90 ml) apple juice

Purple Rain with that smoothie favourite fruit – banana.

NUTRIENTS

Beta-carotene, biotin, folic acid,	ENERGY	★★★★☆
vitamins B1, B2, B5, B6, C and E;	DETOX	★☆☆☆☆
calcium, chromium, iron, magnesium,	IMMUNITY	★★★★☆
manganese, phosphorus, potassium,	DIGESTION	★★★☆☆
sodium, sulphur, zinc; protein	SKIN	★★★★☆

309 | mango in disguise

3 handfuls blueberries and blackberries
1 mango (or 2!)
5 tablespoons (75 ml) natural yogurt
6 tablespoons (90 ml) guava juice

You can barely discern the mango from the colour,
but its taste certainly reminds you it's there, and the
guava adds a different dimension altogether.

NUTRIENTS

Beta-carotene, biotin, folic acid,
vitamins B1, B2, B6, C and E; calcium,
chromium, iron, magnesium, manganese,
phosphorus, potassium, sodium, sulphur,
zinc; protein

ENERGY	★★★★☆
DETOX	★☆☆☆☆
IMMUNITY	★★★★☆
DIGESTION	★★★☆☆
SKIN	★★★★☆

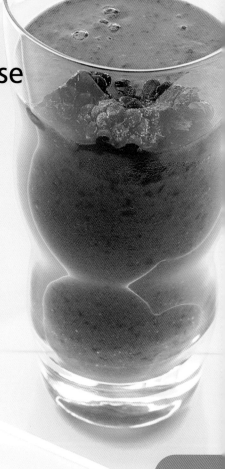

310 | purple pineapple

3 handfuls blueberries, blackberries, blackcurrants
$\frac{1}{2}$ pineapple
5 tablespoons (75 ml) natural yogurt
6 tablespoons (90 ml) pineapple juice

The tangy, tropical taste of pineapple blends beautifully with the berries.
You could even use canned fruits in the winter.

NUTRIENTS

Beta-carotene, biotin, folic acid,
vitamins B1, B2, B6, C and E; calcium,
chromium, iron, magnesium, manganese,
phosphorus, potassium, sodium, sulphur,
zinc; protein

ENERGY	★★★★☆
DETOX	★☆☆☆☆
IMMUNITY	★★★★☆
DIGESTION	★★★☆☆
SKIN	★★★★☆

311 | passionate pine

$\frac{1}{2}$ pineapple
$\frac{1}{2}$ banana
2 passion fruit
5 tablespoons (75 ml) natural yogurt
8 tablespoons (120 ml) pineapple juice

Almost anything with passion fruit is a hit
for me and this is definitely no exception.

NUTRIENTS

Beta-carotene, folic acid, vitamins B1, B3,
B6 and C; calcium, magnesium, manganese,
phosphorus, potassium, sodium, sulphur,
zinc; protein

ENERGY	★★★★☆
DETOX	★☆☆☆☆
IMMUNITY	★★☆☆☆
DIGESTION	★★★★☆
SKIN	★☆☆☆☆

312 | pure pineapple creamy

$\frac{1}{2}$ pineapple
5 tablespoons (75 ml) natural yogurt
8 tablespoons (120ml) pineapple juice

Sometimes the simple ones are the best. Pick a perfectly ripe pineapple
to get the optimum result.

NUTRIENTS

Beta-carotene, folic acid, vitamin C;
calcium, magnesium, manganese,
phosphorus, potassium, sodium,
zinc; protein

ENERGY	★★★★☆
DETOX	★☆☆☆☆
IMMUNITY	★★★☆☆
DIGESTION	★★★★☆
SKIN	★★☆☆☆

313 | pina banana

½ pineapple
2 bananas
2 tablespoons (30 ml) coconut milk
5 tablespoons (75 ml) natural yogurt
6 tablespoons (90 ml) pineapple juice

A truly tropical taste.

NUTRIENTS

Beta-carotene, folic acid, vitamins B1,
B3, B5, B6, C and E; calcium, magnesium,
manganese, phosphorus, potassium,
sodium, sulphur, zinc; protein

ENERGY	★★★★☆
DETOX	★☆☆☆☆
IMMUNITY	★★★☆☆
DIGESTION	★★★☆☆
SKIN	★☆☆☆☆

314 | creamy blue pine

½ pineapple
2 handfuls blueberries
5 tablespoons (75 ml) natural yogurt
8 tablespoons (120 ml) pineapple juice

There's something about the delicious but gentle taste of blueberries
that matches perfectly with tangy pineapple.

NUTRIENTS

Beta-carotene, biotin, folic acid,
vitamins B1, B2, B6, C and E; calcium,
chromium, magnesium, manganese,
phosphorus, potassium, sodium,
zinc; protein

ENERGY	★★★★☆
DETOX	★☆☆☆☆
IMMUNITY	★★★★☆
DIGESTION	★★★★☆
SKIN	★★★★☆

315 | pinkypine

½ pineapple
1 handful strawberries
5 tablespoons (75 ml) natural yogurt
8 tablespoons (120 ml) guava juice

As if the fruit combination wasn't enough to make you salivate,
the guava on top…

NUTRIENTS

Beta-carotene, biotin, folic acid,
vitamin B3, vitamin C; calcium,
magnesium, manganese, phosphorus,
potassium, sodium, sulphur, zinc;
protein

ENERGY	★★★★☆
DETOX	★☆☆☆☆
IMMUNITY	★★★★☆
DIGESTION	★★★☆☆
SKIN	★★★★☆

316 | pure peachy cream

4 peaches
5 tablespoons (75 ml) natural yogurt
8 tablespoons (120 ml) mineral water

Some would ask, why adulterate them with any other fruit?

NUTRIENTS

Beta-carotene, folic acid,
vitamin B3, vitamin C; calcium,
magnesium, phosphorus, potassium,
sodium, sulphur, zinc; protein

ENERGY	★★★★☆
DETOX	★☆☆☆☆
IMMUNITY	★★★★☆
DIGESTION	★★★☆☆
SKIN	★★★☆☆

317 | vanilla peach

3 peaches
1 banana
½ teaspoon vanilla essence
5 tablespoons (75 ml) natural yogurt
8 tablespoons (120 ml) pineapple juice

They're good alone, but most fruits blend well with a banana, the ultimate smoothie fruit.

NUTRIENTS

Beta-carotene, folic acid, vitamins B1,
B3, B6 and C; calcium, magnesium,
phosphorus, potassium, sodium,
sulphur, zinc; protein

ENERGY	★★★★☆
DETOX	★☆☆☆☆
IMMUNITY	★★★☆☆
DIGESTION	★★★★☆
SKIN	★★☆☆☆

318 | peachy passion

2 peaches
¼ pineapple
2 passion fruits
5 tablespoons (75 ml) natural yogurt
8 tablespoons (120 ml) pineapple juice

Another tropical and temperate blend that turns out perfectly.

NUTRIENTS

Beta-carotene, folic acid, vitamin B3,
vitamin C; calcium, iron, magnesium,
manganese, phosphorus, potassium,
sodium, sulphur, zinc; protein

ENERGY	★★★★☆
DETOX	★☆☆☆☆
IMMUNITY	★★★☆☆
DIGESTION	★★★☆☆
SKIN	★★★☆☆

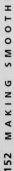

319 | colour blend

2 peaches
1 banana
1 handful raspberries
5 tablespoons (75 ml) natural yogurt
8 tablespoons (120 ml) pineapple juice

Yellow and red make orange – here we have all
three. Best made in the summer with juicy, ripe
peaches and strawberries.

NUTRIENTS

Beta-carotene, biotin, folic acid,
vitamins B1, B3, B6 and C; calcium,
magnesium, phosphorus, potassium,
sodium, sulphur, zinc; protein

ENERGY	★★★★☆
DETOX	★☆☆☆☆
IMMUNITY	★★★☆☆
DIGESTION	★★☆☆☆
SKIN	★★★☆☆

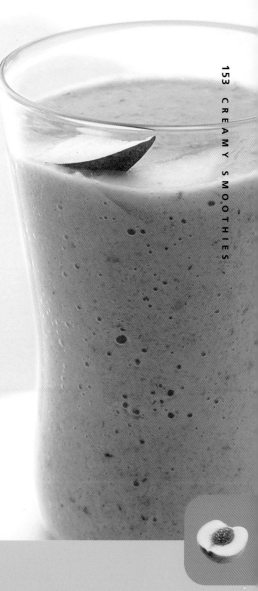

320 | apricot regular

8 rehydrated dried apricots
5 rehydrated prunes
5 tablespoons (75 ml) natural yogurt
8 tablespoons (120 ml) prune juice

Of course you can use any dried fruit, but this one's particularly good
and extremely rich in fibre and antioxidants. It's best to soak the fruit
overnight before blending it.

NUTRIENTS

Beta-carotene, folic acid, vitamins B3, B5
and C; calcium, magnesium, phosphorus,
potassium, sodium, sulphur, zinc; protein

ENERGY	★★★★☆
DETOX	★☆☆☆☆
IMMUNITY	★★★★☆
DIGESTION	★★★★☆
SKIN	★★★★☆

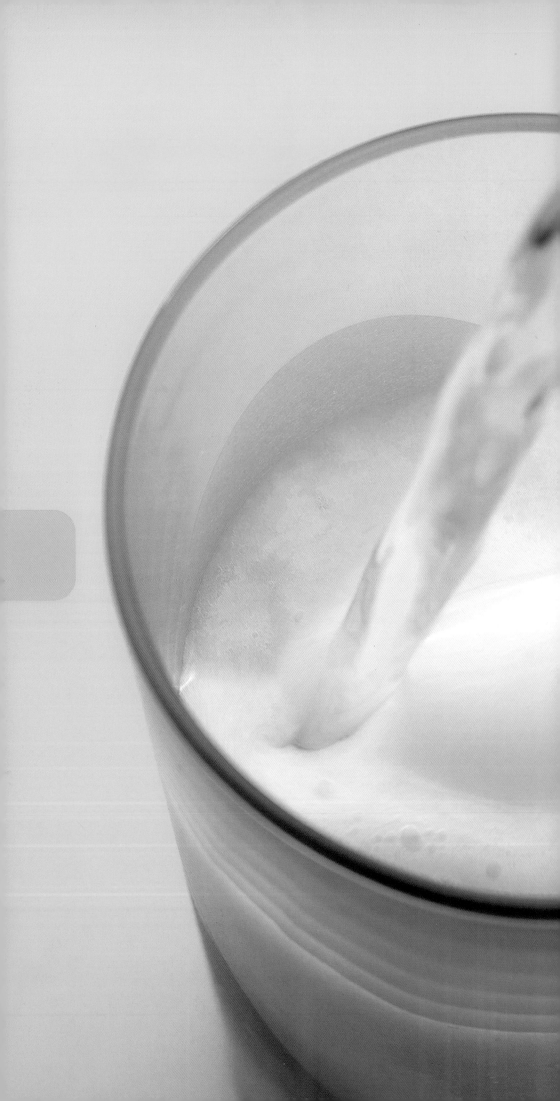

making
quenchers

chapter 4

As if all the other recipes in this book weren't refreshing enough, with quenchers we take that concept to another level. The drinks in this section are largely made with frozen fruit and ice; even the warm teas have a sensationally refreshing taste and texture.

We start with the frozen-fruit quenchers, drinks made by mixing frozen fruit pieces with juices, water, sorbets and ice in a blender to produce delicious combinations, all icy-cold on the palate. Next, the fizzy quenchers are great summer coolers, made by simply mixing all the ingredients (including sparkling mineral water) together in a jug. Finally, the tea-based recipes include home-made blends of warming spices, as well as a selection of cold teas to stimulate and revive the mind and spirit.

Guidelines for making the fizzy and tea-based quenchers are given with each recipe. All of the recipes make two generous portions.

top tips

Below are a few reminders and helpful hints, tips and suggestions to enable you to get the most from making your quenchers.

1   To make frozen-fruit quenchers, drop all of the ingredients into a blender and mix them together for about a minute.

2   To make fizzy quenchers, stir all of the ingredients (including juiced or blended fruit where indicated) together in a large jug.

3   Add some pieces of chopped fruit to your fizzy quenchers to make them more like a summer cocktail.

4   If you want to make a frozen-fruit quencher but are out of frozen fruit, a time-saving alternative is to cheat by using fresh fruit blended with ice.

5   You can make bags of frozen fruit in advance – just prepare the fruit as you would for a smoothie then chop into pieces and divide into convenient sized portions in freezer bags and put in the freezer.

6   To freeze bananas, simply peel them and put them into a freezer bag whole – there is no need to chop them up.

7   When a recipe lists a particular sorbet as one of the ingredients, consider this a suggestion only. Use any sorbet you may have in the freezer – the chances are it'll be delicious whatever you try.

8   Once you've made a few of the recipes, play with the different blends, changing the ingredients to suit your tastes and the contents of your refrigerator, freezer or fruit bowl.

9   With the hot, brewed teas such as Ginger Brew and Full Spice, you can leave the pan on the stove and heat it up later in the day, adding a bit more water and a few more spices. This will deepen the taste and produce a lovely, rich flavour.

10 Most herbs and spices make delicious teas that are also laden with health properties, so try using whatever you've got growing in the garden (or window box), as you're likely to be able to turn it into a refreshing, healthy tea.

321 | tangy banana freeze

2 frozen bananas
1 passion fruit
2 scoops lime sorbet
a few dashes of mineral water

Just blend all of these together for a fresh taste-bomb.

NUTRIENTS

Beta-carotene, folic acid, vitamin B1, B3,
B6 and C; calcium, magnesium, phosphorus,
potassium, sodium, sulphur

ENERGY	★★★★★
DETOX	★☆☆☆☆
IMMUNITY	★★☆☆☆
DIGESTION	★★★☆☆
SKIN	★★★☆☆

322 | orange dream

2 oranges, juiced
4 nectarines
6 ice cubes

This one is like a sweet orange popsicle (ice-lolly) but even better thanks
to the nectarines.

NUTRIENTS

Beta-carotene, folic acid, vitamin C;
calcium, magnesium, phosphorus,
potassium

ENERGY	★★★★★
DETOX	★★☆☆☆
IMMUNITY	★★★★★
DIGESTION	★☆☆☆☆
SKIN	★★★★☆

323 | lift off

2 grapefruits, juiced
$\frac{1}{2}$ pineapple
$\frac{1}{4}$ inch (0.5 cm) grated ginger root
6 ice cubes

This combination is a highly charged challenge to your tastebuds.

NUTRIENTS

Beta-carotene, folic acid, vitamin C;
calcium, magnesium, manganese,
phosphorus, potassium, sodium,
sulphur

ENERGY	★★★★★
DETOX	★☆☆☆☆
IMMUNITY	★★★☆☆
DIGESTION	★★★☆☆
SKIN	★★★☆☆

324 | paw paw sharp

½ papaya
2 scoops lime sorbet
a few dashes of mineral water

I just love the Australian version of papaya – paw paw – and this drink certainly does it justice.

NUTRIENTS

Beta-carotene, folic acid, vitamin C; calcium, magnesium, phosphorus, potassium, sodium, sulphur

ENERGY	★★★★★
DETOX	★☆☆☆☆
IMMUNITY	★★★★☆
DIGESTION	★★★★☆
SKIN	★★★☆☆

325 | mango squeeze

2 grapefruits, juiced
2 mangoes
6 ice cubes

Mango is perfect for toning down the tanginess of the grapefruit – all in all super refreshing and a sweet but uplifting blend.

NUTRIENTS

Beta-carotene, folic acid, vitamin C, vitamin E; calcium, iron, magnesium, phosphorus, potassium, sodium, sulphur

ENERGY	★★★★★
DETOX	★☆☆☆☆
IMMUNITY	★★★★★
DIGESTION	★★☆☆☆
SKIN	★★★★☆

326 | pure pine freeze

½ pineapple, frozen in chunks
1 scoop lime sorbet
a few dashes of pineapple juice

It is hard to imagine anything more thirst quenching than this refreshing drink.

NUTRIENTS

Beta-carotene, folic acid, vitamin C;
calcium, magnesium, manganese,
phosphorus, potassium, sodium,
sulphur

ENERGY	★★★★★
DETOX	★☆☆☆☆
IMMUNITY	★★☆☆☆
DIGESTION	★★★★☆
SKIN	★★★☆☆

327 | pine passion

½ pineapple, frozen in chunks
2 passion fruits
2 tablespoons (30 ml) natural yogurt
a few dashes of pineapple juice

In my view, you can barely go wrong with passion fruit, and blended with frozen, ripe pineapple … mmm.

NUTRIENTS

Beta-carotene, folic acid, vitamins B3,
B12 and C; calcium, iron, magnesium,
manganese, phosphorus, potassium,
sodium, sulphur, zinc; protein

ENERGY	★★★★☆
DETOX	★☆☆☆☆
IMMUNITY	★★★☆☆
DIGESTION	★★★★☆
SKIN	★★★☆☆

328 | tropics at zero

½ pineapple, frozen in chunks
1 mango, frozen in chunks
1 scoop lime sorbet
a few dashes of pineapple juice

You'd certainly need this one on a hot beach in the tropics.

NUTRIENTS

Beta-carotene, folic acid, vitamin C,
vitamin E; calcium, iron, magnesium,
manganese, phosphorus, potassium,
sodium, sulphur

ENERGY	★★★★★
DETOX	★☆☆☆☆
IMMUNITY	★★★★☆
DIGESTION	★★★☆☆
SKIN	★★★★☆

329 | strawberries on sunbeds

$\frac{1}{2}$ pineapple, frozen in chunks
1 handful frozen strawberries
1 tablespoon (15 ml) coconut milk
a few dashes of pineapple juice

Sit back and relax – you'd be forgiven for wondering where in the world
you are with this sublime mix.

NUTRIENTS

Beta-carotene, biotin, folic acid,
vitamin C; calcium, magnesium,
manganese, phosphorus, potassium,
sodium, sulphur

ENERGY	★★★★★
DETOX	★☆☆☆☆
IMMUNITY	★★★★☆
DIGESTION	★★☆☆☆
SKIN	★★★☆☆

330 | malibu freeze

$\frac{1}{2}$ pineapple, frozen in chunks
1 banana, frozen
1 tablespoon (15 ml) coconut milk
$\frac{1}{2}$ lime, juiced
a few dashes of pineapple juice

Transport yourself to beneath a palm tree with this creamy cooler.

NUTRIENTS

Beta-carotene, folic acid, vitamins B1,
B3, B6 and C; calcium, magnesium,
manganese, phosphorus, potassium,
sodium, sulphur

ENERGY	★★★★★
DETOX	★☆☆☆☆
IMMUNITY	★★☆☆☆
DIGESTION	★★★☆☆
SKIN	★★★☆☆

331 | pink banana freeze

2 handfuls frozen strawberries
2 frozen bananas
a few dashes orange juice

A classic smoothie, with a frozen touch.

NUTRIENTS

Beta-carotene, folic acid, biotin,
vitamins B1, B3, B6 and C; calcium,
magnesium, phosphorus, potassium,
sulphur

ENERGY	★★★★★
DETOX	★☆☆☆☆
IMMUNITY	★★★☆☆
DIGESTION	★★☆☆☆
SKIN	★★★☆☆

332 | double red

4 handfuls frozen raspberries
a few dashes cranberry juice

Tangy and sweet all at once, this bright red freezie is exquisite.

NUTRIENTS

Beta-carotene, biotin, folic acid, vitamin C;
calcium, iron, magnesium, manganese,
phosphorus, potassium, sodium, sulphur

ENERGY	★★★★☆
DETOX	★☆☆☆☆
IMMUNITY	★★★☆☆
DIGESTION	☆☆☆☆☆
SKIN	★★★☆☆

333 | double red creamy

2 handfuls frozen raspberries
2 handfuls frozen strawberries
2 tablespoons natural yogurt
a few dashes cranberry juice

A sweeter, creamier version of Double Red, made nice and thick with the
addition of yogurt.

NUTRIENTS

Beta-carotene, biotin, folic acid,
vitamin B12, vitamin C; calcium, iron,
magnesium, manganese, phosphorus,
potassium, sodium, sulphur, zinc,

ENERGY	★★★★☆
DETOX	★☆☆☆☆
IMMUNITY	★★★☆☆
DIGESTION	★★☆☆☆
SKIN	★★★☆☆

334 | peachy pink cream

2 handfuls frozen strawberries
2 peaches, frozen in chunks
2 tablespoons (30 ml) natural yogurt
a few dashes orange juice

An idyllic combination with a creamy touch.

NUTRIENTS

Beta-carotene, biotin, folic acid,
vitamins B3, B12 and C; calcium,
magnesium, phosphorus, potassium,
sodium, sulphur, zinc; protein

ENERGY	★★★★☆
DETOX	★☆☆☆☆
IMMUNITY	★★★★☆
DIGESTION	★★☆☆☆
SKIN	★★★☆☆

335 | big black freeze

4 handfuls frozen blueberries, blackberries, blackcurrants
2 tablespoons (30 ml) natural yogurt
a few dashes apple juice

Whatever the weather, you'd almost believe it was summer when sipping this cooling refresher.

NUTRIENTS

Beta-carotene, biotin, folic acid,
vitamins B1, B2, B6, B12, C and, E;
calcium, chromium, magnesium,
manganese, phosphorus, potassium,
sodium, sulphur, zinc; protein

ENERGY	★★★★☆
DETOX	★☆☆☆☆
IMMUNITY	★★★★★
DIGESTION	★★★☆☆
SKIN	★★★★☆

336 | black & apple freezie

4 handfuls frozen blackberries
2 tablespoons (30 ml) natural yogurt
$\frac{1}{2}$ teaspoon vanilla essence
a few dashes apple juice

That classic English combination with a smooth vanilla undertone.

NUTRIENTS

Beta-carotene, folic acid, vitamin C,
vitamin E; calcium, iron, magnesium,
manganese, phosphorus, potassium,
sodium, sulphur; protein

ENERGY	★★★★☆
DETOX	★☆☆☆☆
IMMUNITY	★★☆☆☆
DIGESTION	☆☆☆☆☆
SKIN	★★★☆☆

337 | creamy apple freezie

4 tablespoons (60 ml) frozen stewed apple
1 fresh apple, cored, chopped and peeled
4 tablespoons (60 ml) natural yogurt
$\frac{1}{4}$ teaspoon ground cinnamon
$\frac{1}{2}$ teaspoon vanilla essence
a few dashes apple juice

This combination is especially good if you've used a sharp variety
of apple such as Granny Smith.

NUTRIENTS

Beta-carotene, folic acid, vitamin B12,
vitamin C; calcium, magnesium, phosphorus,
potassium, sulphur, zinc; protein

ENERGY	★★★★☆
DETOX	★☆☆☆☆
IMMUNITY	★★★☆☆
DIGESTION	★★★★☆
SKIN	★★☆☆☆

338 | gingapple

4 tablespoons (60 ml) frozen stewed apple
2 fresh apples, cored, chopped and peeled
$\frac{1}{4}$ inch (0.5 cm) fresh ginger root, grated
2 scoops lime sorbet
a few dashes apple juice

A deliciously refreshing combination with a sharp bite from the
ginger and lime.

NUTRIENTS

Beta-carotene, folic acid, vitamin C;
calcium, magnesium, phosphorus,
potassium, sodium, sulphur

ENERGY	★★★★☆
DETOX	★☆☆☆☆
IMMUNITY	★★★☆☆
DIGESTION	★★★☆☆
SKIN	★★☆☆☆

339 | pine apple

4 tablespoons (60 ml) frozen stewed apple
$\frac{1}{2}$ pineapple, frozen in chunks
2 scoops lime sorbet
a few dashes apple juice

A wonderfully fresh blend of fruits, given a sweet tang by the
lime sorbet.

NUTRIENTS

Beta-carotene, folic acid, vitamin C;
calcium, magnesium, manganese,
phosphorus, potassium, sodium, sulphur

ENERGY	★★★★☆
DETOX	★☆☆☆☆
IMMUNITY	★★☆☆☆
DIGESTION	★★★☆☆
SKIN	★★☆☆☆

340 | apple & prune freeze

4 tablespoons (60 ml) frozen stewed apple
8 rehydrated prunes
$\frac{1}{2}$ teaspoon vanilla essence
4 tablespoons (60 ml) natural yogurt
a few dashes apple juice

This one is so creamy and sweet – a full meal in itself.

NUTRIENTS

Beta-carotene, folic acid, vitamin B12,
vitamin C; calcium, magnesium, phosphorus,
potassium, sulphur, zinc; protein

ENERGY   ★★★★☆
DETOX   ★☆☆☆☆
IMMUNITY   ★★★★☆
DIGESTION ★★★★☆
SKIN   ★★☆☆☆

341 | blue apple

4 tablespoons (60 ml) frozen stewed apple
2 handfuls frozen blueberries
2 tablespoons (30 ml) natural yogurt
a few dashes apple juice

The flecks of blue from the blueberry skins let you in on the secret
of how delicious this creamy frozen-fruit quencher really is.

NUTRIENTS

Beta-carotene, folic acid, vitamin B12,
vitamin C; calcium, chromium, magnesium,
phosphorus, potassium, sodium, sulphur,
zinc; protein

ENERGY   ★★★★☆
DETOX   ★☆☆☆☆
IMMUNITY   ★★★★☆
DIGESTION ★★★☆☆
SKIN   ★★★★☆

342 | watermelon tanger

$\frac{1}{2}$ watermelon
2 scoops lime sorbet
6 ice cubes

Watermelon is one of the most refreshing fruits, at 95% water, and with the lime added, it's even better. Ideal for a baking hot day.

NUTRIENTS

Beta-carotene, folic acid, vitamin B5, vitamin C; calcium, magnesium, phosphorus, potassium, sodium, sulphur

ENERGY	★★★★★
DETOX	★☆☆☆☆
IMMUNITY	★★★★☆
DIGESTION	☆☆☆☆☆
SKIN	★★★★☆

343 | pink ice

$\frac{1}{2}$ watermelon
2 handfuls frozen strawberries
1 scoop lemon sorbet
6 ice cubes
a few dashes of mineral water

Just by looking at this vision in pink, you'll know it's delicious and good for you.

NUTRIENTS

Beta-carotene, biotin, folic acid, vitamin B5, vitamin C; calcium, magnesium, phosphorus, potassium, sodium, sulphur

ENERGY	★★★★★
DETOX	★☆☆☆☆
IMMUNITY	★★★★☆
DIGESTION	★☆☆☆☆
SKIN	★★★★☆

344 | peachy mango ice

1 mango, frozen in chunks
3 peaches, frozen in chunks
a few dashes of orange juice

Double trouble from two delicious orange fruits that blend beautifully, especially in a frosty drink.

NUTRIENTS

Beta-carotene, folic acid, vitamins B3, C and E; calcium, iron, magnesium, phosphorus, potassium, sodium, sulphur

ENERGY	★★★★★
DETOX	★★☆☆☆
IMMUNITY	★★★★★
DIGESTION	★★☆☆☆
SKIN	★★★★★

345 | mango surprise

2 mangoes, frozen in chunks
juice of one lime
$\frac{1}{2}$ inch (1 cm) grated ginger root
4 tablespoons (60 ml) natural yogurt
6 ice cubes

Your tastebuds won't know what hit them – smooth mango, sharp lime,
zingy ginger and creamy yogurt create a winning combination.

NUTRIENTS

Beta-carotene, folic acid, vitamins B12,
C and E; calcium, iron, magnesium,
phosphorus, potassium, sodium,
sulphur, zinc; protein

ENERGY	★★★★☆
DETOX	★☆☆☆☆
IMMUNITY	★★★☆☆
DIGESTION	★★★☆☆
SKIN	★★★☆☆

346 | apricot banana ice

2 frozen bananas
6 frozen apricots
a few dashes of apple juice

You have to freeze well-ripened apricots to bring out the taste in this
sumptuous quencher; otherwise, freeze apricots that have been canned
in juice.

NUTRIENTS

Beta-carotene, folic acid, vitamins B1,
B3, B5, B6 and C; calcium, magnesium,
phosphorus, potassium, sulphur

ENERGY	★★★★★
DETOX	★☆☆☆☆
IMMUNITY	★★★☆☆
DIGESTION	★★☆☆☆
SKIN	★★★☆☆

347 | kiwi berry

3 kiwi fruits
2 handfuls frozen strawberries
a few dashes of apple juice
4–6 ice cubes

Grab a high dose of vitamin C in this delicious combination.

NUTRIENTS

Beta-carotene, biotin, folic acid,
vitamin C; calcium, magnesium, phosphorus,
potassium, sodium, sulphur

ENERGY	★★★★★
DETOX	★★★☆☆
IMMUNITY	★★★★★
DIGESTION	★★☆☆☆
SKIN	★★★★★

348 | lime cooler

juice of three limes
1 pt (500 ml) sparkling mineral water
4–6 fresh mint leaves
4–6 ice cubes

A classic, cooling summer drink, perfect in its simplicity.

NUTRIENTS

Beta-carotene, folic acid, vitamin C;	ENERGY	★☆☆☆☆
calcium, magnesium, phosphorus,	DETOX	★★☆☆☆
potassium, sodium, sulphur	IMMUNITY	★★★☆☆
	DIGESTION	★☆☆☆☆
	SKIN	★★☆☆☆

349 | orange passion twinkle

4 oranges, juiced
4 passion fruits
sparkling mineral water to top up
4–6 ice cubes

Perfect on a hot summer's day, just stir in the passion fruit. If you don't
like the seeds, pass them through a strainer first.

NUTRIENTS

Beta-carotene, vitamin B3, vitamin C;	ENERGY	★★★★☆
calcium, magnesium, phosphorus,	DETOX	★★☆☆☆
potassium, sodium	IMMUNITY	★★★★☆
	DIGESTION	☆☆☆☆☆
	SKIN	★★☆☆☆

350 | grape cooler

2 grapefruits, juiced
1 scoop orange sorbet
$\frac{1}{4}$ inch (0.5 cm) grated ginger root
sparkling mineral water to top up
4–6 ice cubes

Just let the sorbet melt, sweeten and froth up the freshly squeezed
juice before splashing in the mineral water to give it fizz.

NUTRIENTS

Beta-carotene, folic acid, vitamin C;	ENERGY	★★★★☆
calcium, magnesium, phosphorus,	DETOX	★★☆☆☆
potassium, sulphur	IMMUNITY	★★★★☆
	DIGESTION	★☆☆☆☆
	SKIN	★★☆☆☆

351 | pine fizz

½ pineapple, juiced
4–6 fresh mint leaves
sparkling mineral water to top up
4–6 ice cubes

Somehow, pineapples really suit being fizzy.

NUTRIENTS

Beta-carotene, folic acid, vitamin C;
calcium, magnesium, manganese,
phosphorus, potassium, sodium

ENERGY	★★★★☆
DETOX	★★★☆☆
IMMUNITY	★★★☆☆
DIGESTION	★★★☆☆
SKIN	★★☆☆☆

352 | pick-me-up fizz

½ pineapple, juiced
2 oranges, juiced
sparkling mineral water to top up
4–6 ice cubes

Fresh, tangy, sharp, juicy, fizzy – all sensations to liven you up.

NUTRIENTS

Beta-carotene, folic acid, vitamin C;
calcium, magnesium, manganese,
phosphorus, potassium, sodium

ENERGY	★★★★☆
DETOX	★★☆☆☆
IMMUNITY	★★★★☆
DIGESTION	★★☆☆☆
SKIN	★★★☆☆

353 | melon tang

1 melon
¼ inch (0.5 cm) grated ginger root
juice of a lime
4–6 ice cubes
sparkling mineral water to top up

Blend the melon, lime juice, ginger and ice before topping up
to a fizzy cooler.

NUTRIENTS

Beta-carotene, folic acid, vitamin C;
calcium, magnesium, phosphorus,
potassium, sodium, sulphur

ENERGY	★★★★☆
DETOX	★★☆☆☆
IMMUNITY	★★★☆☆
DIGESTION	★★☆☆☆
SKIN	★★★☆☆

354 | fizzy berry crush

2 handfuls strawberries
2 handfuls blueberries
4–6 ice cubes
sparkling mineral water to top up

Instead of fruit juice, use fruit pulp by blending
the strawberries and blueberries with the ice, so
you get a fantastic texture as well as taste.

NUTRIENTS

Beta-carotene, biotin, folic acid,
vitamins B1, B2, B6, C and E; calcium,
chromium, magnesium, phosphorus,
potassium, sodium, sulphur

ENERGY	★★★★☆
DETOX	★★★☆☆
IMMUNITY	★★★★★
DIGESTION	☆☆☆☆☆
SKIN	★★★★☆

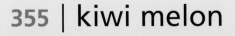

355 | kiwi melon

$\frac{1}{2}$ melon
2 kiwi fruits
juice of a lime
4–6 ice cubes
sparkling mineral water to top up

Another blended fizzie – pulp the melon, kiwi, lime juice and ice
before adding the mineral water for a delicious summery cocktail.

NUTRIENTS

Beta-carotene, folic acid, vitamin C;
calcium, magnesium, phosphorus,
potassium, sodium, sulphur

ENERGY	★★★★☆
DETOX	★★★☆☆
IMMUNITY	★★★★★
DIGESTION	★☆☆☆☆
SKIN	★★★★☆

356 | apple spice

$\frac{1}{2}$ inch (0.5 cm) grated or finely sliced ginger root
2 cinnamon sticks
7 fl oz (200 ml) water
1 teaspoon honey
4 tablespoons frozen stewed apple
7 fl oz (200 ml) apple juice

This is a delicious blend of apples and spices in a summer drink. Alternatively, you could drink it warm on a cold winter's night.

Bring the water, ginger and cinnamon to the boil and leave to simmer for at least five minutes. Strain, add the honey and leave to cool. Meanwhile, mix the apple and apple juice in a blender and gradually add the cooled tea.

357 | fresh sensation

1 small bunch of fresh mint leaves
1 inch (2.5 cm) grated ginger root
9 fl oz (300 ml) water
4 oranges, freshly juiced
1 scoop lime sorbet
4–6 ice cubes

A combination of refreshing, tangy ingredients to cool down on a summer's day.

Pour boiling water over the leaves and grated ginger, steep for five minutes. Leave to cool, top up with freshly squeezed orange juice, lime sorbet and ice.

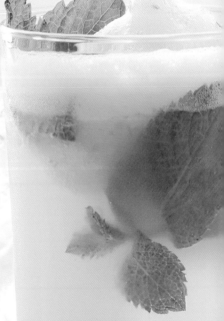

358 | ginger brew

1 inch (2.5 cm) grated ginger root
1 pt (500 ml) water

Neat ginger tea, refreshing and good for digestion.
If you find it a little strong-tasting, add a teaspoon
of honey for a more mellow flavour.

Bring to the boil and leave to simmer for at least five minutes.
Strain and serve.

359 | middle east ginger

1 inch (2.5 cm) grated ginger root
10 cardamom pods
1 pt (500 ml) water

Ginger Brew with a touch of the Middle East from the
cardamom, even better for digestion.

Bring to the boil and leave to simmer for at least five minutes.
Strain and serve.

360 | cold soother

2 sticks cinnamon
juice of a lemon
1 teaspoon honey
1 pt (500 ml) water

A warm drink to soothe the throat on a winter's day.

Bring water and cardamom to the boil and leave to simmer for at
least five minutes. Strain, add the lemon juice and honey and serve.

361 | full spice

$\frac{1}{2}$ inch (1 cm) grated or finely sliced ginger root
4 cardamom pods
1 cinnamon stick
5 cloves
1 pt (500 ml) water

A complete blend of delicious spices for a warming
drink that's great for soothing the throat and digestion.

Bring to the boil and leave to simmer for at least five minutes.
Strain and serve.

362 | mint & honey

1 small bunch of fresh mint leaves
1 teaspoon honey
1 pt (500 ml) water

Fresh mint tea is probably the most refreshing hot drink there
is, and it's good for digestion. I don't usually add honey, but to
make it more like the sweet Middle Eastern version, you can stir
in a spoonful.

Pour boiling water over the leaves, steep for five minutes. If using honey, stir
it in and serve.

363 | tangy mint cooler

1 small bunch of fresh mint leaves
9 fl oz (300 ml) water
7 fl oz (200 ml) pineapple juice
4–6 ice cubes

A refreshing minty cocktail to stimulate the senses.

Make mint tea as in Mint & Honey (see above), leave to cool. Top up with
pineapple juice and add ice.

364 | rosehip rasp

1 rosehip teabag
14 fl oz (400 ml) water
1 handful raspberries
2 peaches, frozen in chunks
4–6 ice cubes

Rosehip tea has a sharp, fruity, refreshing taste –
the fruit contrasts with this perfectly and gives your
immune system an extra boost.

Pour boiling water over the teabag. Leave to steep and cool.
Meanwhile, blend the raspberries and peach. Stir the fruit pulp
into the cooled tea and add ice cubes.

365 | spicy peachy cream

4 cardamom pods
2 cinnamon sticks
7 fl oz (200 ml) water
3 peaches, frozen in chunks
$\frac{1}{2}$ teaspoon vanilla essence
3 tablespoons (45 ml) natural yogurt
3–5 ice cubes

This one is almost a dessert in itself – a
fantastic blend of eastern spices, fresh peaches
and creamy yogurt.

Bring the water, cardamom and cinnamon
to the boil and leave to simmer for at least
five minutes. Strain and leave to cool. Meanwhile
mix the peaches, vanilla and yogurt in blender
and gradually add the spice tea. Top with
ice cubes and sip slowly through a straw.

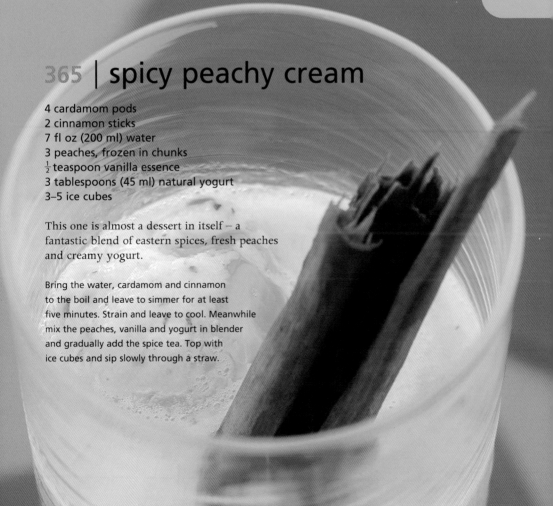

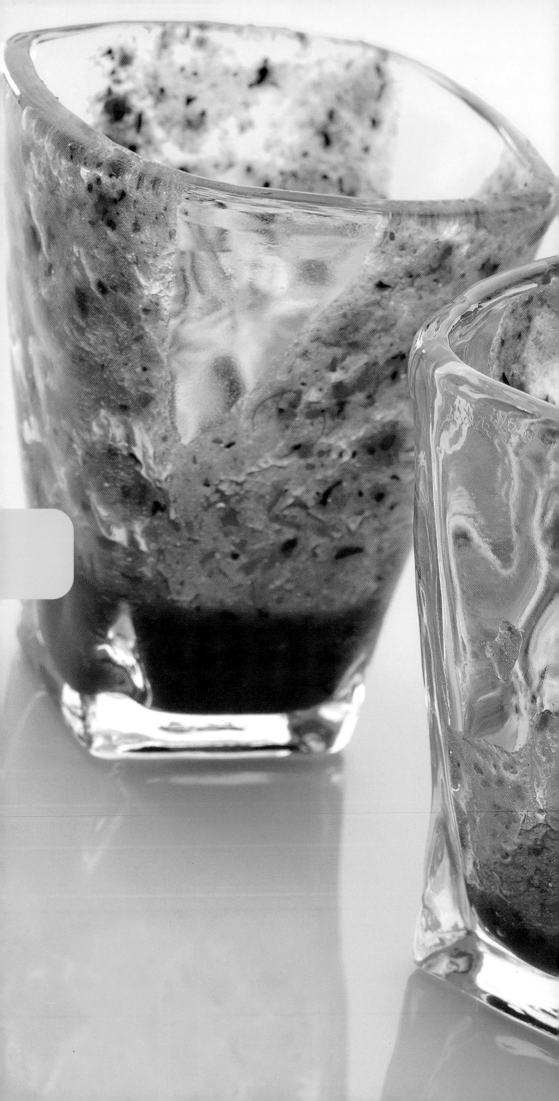

juicing
reference
chapter 5

This section starts with four healthful programs to make choosing your juice recipes easy. If you're just getting into the habit, begin with The Basic Intro Week, to start you off gently on simple, delicious fruit and vegetable drinks. Then there's The Detox Week: juices chosen to accompany a basic detox program. If you tend to get every cough and cold going, you'd do well to give your immune system a boost by having a daily, fresh juice as suggested in The Immune Power Week. Finally, the last juice course is a wonderfully rejuvenating Juice High Weekend, where, for nearly 48 hours, you feast on nothing but juices.

Following on from the juice courses, you'll find two useful charts: a list of nutrients, what they're good for and rich food sources, then an easy reference of fruits, vegetables and juice recipes to help support you for a number of common ailments.

the basic intro week

To inspire you through the maze of the countless combinations possible, this starter course introduces you to some juice recipes that are likely to become your staples. Working primarily with ingredients that you're most likely to have in your fruit bowl or refrigerator, we build up from simple fruit juices to blends you may initially have found a little challenging on the palate. Believe me, if you're not already, by the time you've got to the end of this week, you'll be a true juicing devotee.

Monday	Sweet C Too (see p.31)
Tuesday	Pink Pear (see p.67)
Wednesday	Gently Raspberry (see p.58)
Thursday	Pineapple Basic (see p.73)
Friday	Orange Carrot (see p.78)
Saturday	Easy Morning (see p.77)
Sunday	Apple Cleanser (see p.33)

the detox week

Many health-conscious people occasionally "go on a detox". First, it's important to remember that our bodies are constantly detoxifying, not just when we choose. Second, some of the faddy programs are, in my view, too extreme and in some cases unhealthy. However, others programs encourage us to reassess what we are consuming, and leave us feeling rejuvenated, clearer in mind and body and bursting with energy. The recipes here are particularly cleansing blends aimed at supporting you during a sensible detox program.

Monday	Apple Cleanser (see p.33)
Tuesday	Green Hit (see p.83)
Wednesday	Carrot Cleanser (see p.78)
Thursday	Beet Basic (see p.95)
Friday	Green Goddess (see p.91)
Saturday	Green 'n' Pear It (see p.91)
Sunday	Green Pines (see p.75)

the immune-power week

If you've noticed that your body's defences are not up to scratch – you pick up any passing cold and regularly suffer from throat or bladder infections – your immune system may need a hand. Even if you've always had a tendency to get ill, you should find that giving yourself a boost with fresh, raw juices and smoothies helps keep colds at bay, let alone anything more serious. These recipes are particularly powerful immune-boosters for a concerted one-week course, but you'll feel even more benefit if you make juicing an ongoing delight.

Monday	Power Packed C (see p.49)
Tuesday	Carotene Kick (see p.97)
Wednesday	Cold War (see p.81)
Thursday	Grapefruit Blues (see p.42)
Friday	Greatfruit C (see p.42)
Saturday	Carotene Catapult (see p.80)
Sunday	Green Tomatoes (see p.100)

the juice high weekend

By consuming nothing but raw, fresh juices for a weekend, you give your body a break from the foods and drinks that normally travel through your insides. This way, the body has a chance to do a bit of its own housework and leave you rejuvenated and feeling like you're making a fresh start. It is also a good step in helping you kick a toxic habit such as smoking. This may not sound like a huge amount of fun, and it is likely to be challenging, so it's best to go on a juice fast over a weekend or two-day break, when you can relax and rest as you feel is necessary.

You'll find you get the most out of this course if you prepare yourself well beforehand by buying in all you need, and see it as treating yourself to two days of healthy calm. In addition to drinking the blends listed overleaf (about 6 glasses a day in total), I suggest you incorporate the following into your weekend: plenty of spring water, several snoozes (you may feel tired, irritable or get a bit of a headache), a sauna or steam, a warm bath (spinkle in a few drops of your favourite essential oils), a massage, gentle walks in fresh air, breathing exercises, and pastimes, such as reading, to keep you busy if you are not sleeping. Avoid strenuous exercise.

Day Before	Eat light salads and fruit during the day.	
	Dinner	Green Hit (see p.83)

Day One	Breakfast	Apple Gone Loupey (see p.36)
	Late morning	Florida Blue (see p.48)
	Afternoon	Beetles (see p.95)
	Dinner	Green Goddess (see p.91)

Day Two	Breakfast	Carrot Deep Cleanser (see p.79)
	Mid-morning	Beet Basic (see p.95)
	Lunch	Large salad of fresh, raw vegetables and/or fruits.
	Dinner	Large salad of fresh, raw vegetables and/or fruits.

It is crucial that you do not suddenly overload your body with large quantities of cooked or rich foods. Prepare a substantial, varied salad and dress it lightly with olive oil and lemon juice. Sit down to eat it and chew it well.

Most people are likely to feel a little tired doing the Juice High Weekend. You may also experience some bloating or flatulence, diarrhea, headaches, tiredness and sweating. These are normal; however, if they become excessive or you have other symptoms, you should visit a doctor. You should not undertake the Juice High Weekend if you are unwell, pregnant or on medication.

nutrient chart

This chart lists the main nutrients that the body needs for optimum health. The right-hand column gives all the rich food sources for each nutrient – including foods that are not used in juices or smoothies but that should nevertheless form part of your regular diet.

nutrient	benefits	rich food sources
vitamins		
Vitamin A	Important antioxidant, protects skin and keeps vision healthy; protects against cancer.	Butter, kidneys, liver, whole milk
Beta-carotene	Important antioxidant, protects skin – including "inside skins" such as the lining of intestines, lungs, nose and throat. Beta-carotene is the plant version of vitamin A.	Apricots, asparagus, broccoli, cantaloupe melon, carrots, kale, liver, pumpkin, spinach, sweet potato, watermelon
Vitamin B1 (thiamine)	Needed for energy production; and for the normal workings of the nervous system, muscles and heart, growth and development.	Beef kidney and liver, brewer's yeast, chickpeas, kidney beans, rice bran, salmon, soy (soya) beans, sunflower seeds, wheatgerm, whole grain wheat and rye
Vitamin B2 (riboflavin)	Needed for the production of energy from food, and for healthy skin and mucous membranes; needed for nerves to function well and for healthy growth and development.	Almonds, brewer's yeast, cheese, chicken, eggs, fish, milk, organic meats, wheatgerm, yogurt
Vitamin B3 (niacin)	Needed for the production of energy, the health of the nervous system, digestive system and skin; also needed to keep cholesterol levels low.	Beef liver, brewer's yeast, chicken, fish, nuts, potatoes, pulses, sunflower seeds, turkey
Vitamin B5 (pantothenic acid)	Needed for energy production, the body's response to stress, regeneration of all of cells, particularly in the nervous system, and antibodies.	Blue cheese, brewer's yeast, corn, dried fruit, eggs, lentils, liver, lobster, meat, nuts, peas, soy (soya) beans, sunflower seeds, wheatgerm, whole grain products, vegetables
Vitamin B6 (pyridoxine)	Needed for energy production, a healthy nervous system, brain and mental state, and for the body to build all types of cells, hormones and anti-bodies (defenders against infections).	Avocados, bananas, bran, brewer's yeast, carrots, eggs, hazelnuts, lean meat, lentils, rice, salmon, shrimps, soy (soya) beans, sunflower seeds, tuna, wheatgerm, wholewheat flour
Vitamin B12 (cyanocobalamin)	Particularly important for the health of the brain and nervous system and for formation of red blood cells.	Cheese, clams, eggs, fish, meat, milk and milk products, poultry. NB – vitamin B12 is not found in plant foods.
Folic acid	Needed for production of red blood cells, and the growth of healthy nerves, particularly in a developing fetus.	Barley, brewer's yeast, fruit, chickpeas, green leafy vegetables, lentils, liver, peas, rice, soy (soya) beans, wheatgerm
Biotin	Helps the body process sugars, carbohydrates, proteins and other vitamins; needed for healthy skin, nails and hair.	Brewer's yeast, brown rice, cashew nuts, cheese, chicken, eggs, lentils, liver, mackerel, meat, milk, oats, peanuts, peas, soy (soya) beans, sunflower seeds, tuna, walnuts

nutrient	benefits	rich food sources
Vitamin C (ascorbic acid)	Countless uses: promotes healthy blood capillaries and gums, and healthy skin and healing; aids absorption of iron and production of hemoglobin; boosts the body's defences against illnesses, helps protect against cancer, heart disease, allergies, infections, colds, stress and even aging.	Blackcurrants, broccoli, Brussels sprouts, grapefruit, green bell pepper, guava, kale, kiwi fruits, lemons, oranges, papayas, potatoes, spinach, strawberries, tomatoes, watercress
Vitamin D	Helps control use of calcium, needed for strong bones and teeth.	Cod liver oil, eggs, herring, mackerel, salmon, sardines
Vitamin E	Antioxidant; helps protect skin, circulation, brain, hormones and much more against effects of pollution; anti-clotting properties protect against heart disease.	Almonds, corn oil, hazelnuts, sunflower seeds and oil, walnuts, wheatgerm, wholewheat flour
Vitamin K	Needed to ensure the blood can clot normally.	Broccoli, Brussels sprouts, green cabbage, spinach, Camembert cheese, cauliflower, Cheddar cheese, green tea, oats, soy (soya) beans
minerals		
Calcium	Best-known for building healthy bones, so particularly important for growing children and women reaching menopause at risk of osteoporosis. Also needed for muscles to contract and relax properly (including the heart muscle) and for healthy nerve function.	Almonds, Brazil nuts, cheese, green leafy vegetables, kelp, milk, molasses, salmon (canned), sardines (canned), sesame seeds, shrimp, soy (soya) beans, yogurt
Chromium	Helps processing of sugars and carbohydrates; works with the hormone insulin to balance blood sugar levels and hence, energy, concentration and appetite.	Beef, brewer's yeast, cheese, chicken, eggs, fish, fruit, liver, molasses, potatoes, seafood, whole grains
Copper	Needed in tiny amounts in the body for proper transport and production of red blood cells, and for triggering the release of iron to form hemoglobin.	Barley, cocoa, honey, lentils, molasses, mushrooms, mussels, nuts, oats, oysters, salmon, seeds, wheatgerm
Iodine	Forms part of the thyroid hormone that controls metabolism.	Cod liver oil, fish, oysters, table salt (iodized), seaweed, sunflower seeds
Iron	Part of hemoglobin – the red blood cell substance which carries oxygen from the lungs around the body to all the cells. Also needed as a catalyst for other processes in the body including cell reproduction.	Cashew nuts, cheese, egg yolks, chickpeas, green leafy vegetables, lean meat, lentils, molasses, mussels, offal, pumpkin seeds, sardines, seaweed, walnuts, wheatgerm
Magnesium	Works with calcium in many body functions, such as the transmission of messages down nerve cells, contraction and relaxation of muscles, growth and development of bones; also for the production of energy.	Almonds, fish, green leafy vegetables, molasses, nuts, soy (soya) beans, sesame and sunflower seeds, wheatgerm

nutrient	benefits	rich food sources
Manganese	An antioxidant, needed for healthy nerves and brain, and sex hormone production.	Avocados, barley, blackberries, brown rice, buckwheat, chestnuts, ginger, hazelnuts, oats, peas, pecans, seaweed, spinach
Potassium	Works with sodium to control normal nerve function and muscle contraction, including a regular heartbeat. The two also help balance the flow of water and nutrients in and out of cells preventing water retention.	Avocados, bananas, citrus fruits, lentils, milk, molasses, nuts, parsnips, potatoes, raisins, sardines (canned), spinach, whole grains
Selenium	Works with vitamin E as a powerful antioxidant to protect against degenerative diseases including certain cancers, heart disease and aging.	Avocados, broccoli, cabbage, celery, chicken, egg yolks, garlic, lentils, liver, milk, mushrooms, onions, seafood, wheatgerm, whole grains
Sodium	Alongside potassium, helps control the water balance in the body. Important for regulating blood pressure, healthy nervous function and normal muscle contraction and relaxation.	Table salt and most commercially processed and packaged foods, as well as bacon, bread, butter, ham, milk, canned vegetables
Sulphur	Antioxidant; also helps the liver release bile and detoxify various substances; needed for the production of collagen, our cellular "glue", so it is important for skin health and the repair of injured skin.	Cabbage, clams, eggs, fish, garlic, milk, onions, wheatgerm
Zinc	Acts as an antioxidant; is needed for normal taste; also needed for the growth and regeneration of new cells (particularly important in fetal development and teenagers); helps skin heal; needed for healthy reproductive organs, especially in men.	Egg yolks, fish, milk, molasses, oysters, peanuts, red meat, sesame seeds, soy (soya) beans, sunflower seeds, turkey, wheatgerm, whole grains
other important nutrients		
Essential fatty acids	Needed for brain power, healthy nerves, smooth skin, hormone balance and more, these fats are incorporated into the membrane or skin of every cell in the body to keep each one working optimally.	Fish such as herring, mackerel, salmon and sardines; nuts; seeds such as hemp, flaxseeds, pumpkin, sesame and sunflower
Protein	Forms the basic material of all living cells – not just thoses that form the structure of our bodies but also blood cells, hormones and much more. Dietary sources are essential for rebuilding and regeneration, and for all body systems to function.	Eggs, fish, meat, milk, poultry, soy (soya)

juices for ailments

This chart lists the best foods to eat to help your body fight a range of common ailments, and offers a selection of the juice recipes that are rich in such foods. However, drinking the juices suggested is intended as a supplement to, and not a replacement for, professional medical advice.

ailment	foods to eat	no.	juice title
Acne	All greens (such as broccoli, kale, parsley, spinach, watercress), fruit and vegetable fibre, garlic, seeds and their oils, yogurt	172 175 257 310	Green Waldorf Super Defender Heaven Scent Purple Pineapple
Anemia	All greens (such as broccoli, kale, parsley, spinach, watercress), beets (beetroot), berries, kiwi fruit, citrus fruit, molasses	176 189 180 066	Grape & Green Tabouleh Beetles Blackcurrant Twist
Angina	Broccoli, citrus fruis, fruit and vegetable fibre, kale, kiwi fruit, seeds and their oils, strawberries, watercress, wheatgerm	169 172 245 258	Green 'n' Pear It Green Waldorf Mango Blues Globe Trotter
Arthritis	Apricots, berries; broccoli, carrots, garlic, ginger, kiwi fruit, mango, pineapple, red bell pepper, seeds and their oils, watercress, wheatgerm	111 127 156 082	Breakfast Pear Joint Aid Carrot Joint Aid Berry Bonanza
Asthma	Apricots, berries, broccoli, carrots, ginger, kale, mango, melon, red bell pepper, seeds and their oils, sweet potato, watercress, watermelon	120 177 135 261	Ginger Zinger Creamy Green Carrot Crunch Peachy Strawbs
Bladder problems	Blueberries, broccoli, citrus fruit, cranberries, garlic, kiwi fruit, strawberries, watermelon, yogurt	028 137 267 276	Cranapple Carotene Catapult Cranapple Crush Watermelon Crush
Boils	All greens (such as broccoli, kale, parsley, spinach, watercress), berries, citrus fruits, fruit and vegetable fibre, garlic, kiwi fruits	071 168 134 242	Orange Pepper Green Apple Carrot Deep Cleanser Summer Mango Special
Bronchitis	Apricots, broccoli, carrots, citrus fruit, garlic, kale, kiwi fruit, mango, melon, red bell pepper, seeds and their oils, strawberries, sweet potato, watercress, watermelons	039 117 141 137	Greatfruit C Black Pineapple Cold War Carotene Catapult
Burns, cuts & bruises	Apricots, broccoli, cabbage, carrots, citrus fruit, garlic, kale, kiwi fruit, mango, milk, red bell pepper, seeds and their oils, strawberries, watercress, yogurt	054 065 259 295	Bright Orange Muddy Puddle Supreme Strawberry Pinky Mango
Bursitis	Apricots, broccoli, cabbage, carrots, citrus fruit, garlic, ginger, kale, kiwi fruit, mango, pineapple, red bell pepper, seeds and their oils, strawberries, watercress	120 127 078 262	Ginger Zinger Joint Aid Sharp Citrusberry Pink Berry Crush
Candidiasis	All greens (such as broccoli, kale, parsley, spinach, watercress), yogurt	169 134 140 312	Green 'n' Pear It Carrot Deep Cleanser Veggie Carotene Catapult Pure Pineapple Creamy

ailment	foods to eat	no.	juice title
Cardiovascular disease	Broccoli, citrus fruit, fruit and vegetable fibre, kale, kiwi fruit, seeds and their oils, strawberries, watercress, wheatgerm	057 057 127 217 259	Power Packed C Joint Aid Take Heart Supreme Strawberry
Chronic catarrh	Apricots, berries, carrots, citrus fruit, mango, melon, papaya, pineapple, watermelon	136 149 117 257	Carrot Digestif Florida Carrot Black Pineapple Heaven Scent
Chronic fatigue	All greens (such as broccoli, kale, parsley, spinach, watercress), bananas, berries, citrus fruit, kale, kiwi fruit, seeds and their oils, watercress, wheatgerm, yogurt	164 167 285 306	Salad Cooler Green Goddess Green Banana Creamy Purple Rain
Cold sores	Apricots, berries, broccoli, carrots, citrus fruit, garlic, kale, kiwi fruit, mango, red bell pepper, strawberries, tomatoes, watercress	057 141 140 194	Power Packed C Cold War Veggie Carotene Catapult Green Tomatoes
Colitis	Apples, apricots, broccoli, cabbage, carrots, citrus fruit, fruit and vegetable fibre, kale, kiwi fruit, mango, melon, papaya, pineapple, seeds and seed oils, strawberries, watercress, wheatgerm	012 140 173 254	Apple Cleanser Veggie Carotene Catapult Sweet Green Melon Papaya Pure
Common cold & 'flu	Apricots, broccoli, carrots, citrus fruit, garlic, ginger, kale, kiwi fruit, mango, melon, nectarines, red bell pepper, strawberries, watercress, watermelons	057 141 244 263	Power Packed C Cold War Nectargo Citrus Strawbs
Constipation	Fruit and vegetable fibre, plenty of water and juices, seeds and their oils	002 180 235 320	Apple Basic Beetles Regular Banana Apricot Regular
Cough	Apricots, berries, broccoli, carrots, citrus fruit, garlic, ginger, kale, kiwi fruit, mango, melon, papaya, pineapple, red bell pepper, sweet potato, watercress, watermelon	040 117 137 255	Surprising Sweetie Black Pineapple Carotene Catapult Papaya Salad
Cystitis	Broccoli, citrus fruit, cranberries, garlic, kiwi fruit, strawberries, pineapple, watermelon, yogurt	028 267 276 315	Cranapple Cranapple Crush Watermelon Crush Pinkypine
Dermatitis	Apples, apricots, berries, broccoli, carrots, celery, citrus fruit, garlic, kale, kiwi fruit, mango, melon, red bell pepper, seeds and their oils, watercress, watermelon	022 133 205	Apple Gone Loupey Carrot Cleanser Creamy Crunch Any juice/smoothie with added seed oil
Diabetes	All greens (such as broccoli, kale, parsley, spinach, watercress), fruit and vegetable fibre, seeds and their oils	136 176 175 252	Carrot Digestif Grape & Green Super Defender Pineberry

ailment	foods to eat	no.	juice title
Diarrhea	Apples, carrots, celery, pears	001	Eve's Downfall
		027	Apple Zing
		100	Pear Basic
		205	Creamy Crunch
Diverticulitis	Fruit and vegetable fibre, garlic, ginger, yogurt	004	Basic with a Boost
		126	Digestaid
		258	Globe Trotter
		312	Pure Pineapple Creamy
Dry skin	Apricots, berries, broccoli, carrots, citrus fruit, garlic, kale, kiwi fruit, mango, melon, red bell pepper, seeds and their oils, watercress, watermelon	149	Florida Carrot
		082	Berry Bonanza
			Any juice/smoothie with added seeds/seed oil
Ear infection	Apricots, berries, broccoli, carrots, citrus fruit, garlic, kale, kiwi fruit, mango, melon, red bell pepper, seeds and their oils, watercress, watermelon	070	Water Cooler II
		141	Cold War
		140	Veggie Carotene Catapult
		082	Berry Bonanza
Eczema	Berries, broccoli, carrots, garlic, kale, kiwi fruit, mango, melon, red bell pepper, seeds and their oils, watercress, watermelon	127	Joint Aid
		137	Carotene Catapult
		177	Creamy Green
		265	Blue Healer
Endometriosis	All fruit and vegetable juice and fibre, seeds and their oils, soy (soya) milk, yogurt	069	Orange Aniseed Twist
		133	Carrot Cleanser
		253	Apple Squared
			Any smoothie with soy (soya) milk
Eyesight Problems	Apricots, berries, carrots, kale, mango, melon, pineapple, red bell pepper, watercress, watermelon	129	What's Up Doc?
		155	Capple and Black
		265	Blue Healer
		314	Blue Pine Creamy
Fatigue	All fruit and vegetable juice and fibre, bananas, berries, carrots, pears, molasses, yogurt	111	Breakfast Pear
		133	Carrot Cleanser
		285	Green Banana Creamy
		307	Mighty Berry
Fever	All fresh fruit and vegetable juices (especially apricots, berries, broccoli, carrots, citrus fruit, kale, kiwi fruit, mango, melon, red bell pepper, sweet potato, watercress, watermelon), garlic, seeds and their oils	059	Orange Medley
		141	Cold War
		185	Carotene Kick
		275	Pure Watermelon
Fibroids	All greens (such as broccoli, kale, parsley, spinach, watercress), celery, citrus fruit, fennel, fruit and vegetable fibre, pears, soy (soya) milk, seeds and their oils	069	Orange Aniseed Twist
		169	Green 'n' Pear It
			Any smoothie with soya milk and seeds/seed oil
Food poisoning	Apples, carrots, celery, ginger, pears	002	Eve's Downfall
		027	Apple Zing
		100	Pear Basic
		205	Creamy Crunch

ailment	foods to eat	no.	juice title
Fractures	All greens (such as broccoli, kale, parsley, spinach, watercress), milk, molasses, peaches, pineapple, seeds and their oils, soy (soya) milk, yogurt	065	Muddy Puddle
		167	Green Goddess
		290	Peachy Banana Dream
		314	Creamy Blue Pine
Gallbladder disorders	Apples, beet (beetroot), grapefruit, yogurt	133	Carrot Cleanser
		180	Beetles
		181	Blood 'n' Grape
		166	Bloody Cuke
Gout	Cabbage, carrots, celery, cherries, kale, strawberries	094	Cherry Pie
		098	Cherry Cooler
		145	Carrot Lift
		214	Soft and Sharp
Hemorrhoids	Apricots, berries, broccoli, carrots, citrus fruit, fruit and vegetable fibre, kale, kiwi fruit, mango, melon, red bell pepper, watercress, watermelon, wheatgerm	016	Black Orchard Berry Buster
		055	Florida Blue
		155	Capple and Black
		250	Pastel Perfect
Hangovers	All greens (such as broccoli, kale, parsley, spinach, watercress), apples, bananas, carrots, celery, ginger, yogurt	027	Apple Zing
		133	Carrot Cleanser
		277	Creamy Cooler
		285	Green Banana Creamy
Hay fever	Apricots, berries, broccoli, carrots, citrus fruit, kale, kiwi fruit, mango, melon, seeds and their oils, strawberries, sweet potato, watercress, watermelon	057	Power Packed C
		171	Green Grapefruit
		137	Carotene Catapult
		259	Supreme Strawberry
Heartburn	Cabbage, papaya, pineapple	030	Bellyful
		113	Gut Soother
		126	Digestaid
		254	Papaya Pure
Herpes	Berries, broccoli, carrots, citrus fruit, garlic, kale, kiwi fruit, seeds and their oils, tomatoes, watercress	057	Power Packed C
		141	Cold War
		140	Veggie Carotene Catapult
		194	Green Tomatoes
High blood pressure	All fresh fruit and vegetables, especially greens (such as broccoli, kale, parsley, spinach, watercress), apples, garlic, seeds and their oils, wheatgerm	022	Apple Gone Loupey
		147	Green Hit
		214	Soft and Sharp
		217	Take Heart
Hives (Urticaria)	Apricots, berries, broccoli, carrots, citrus fruit, garlic, kale, kiwi fruit, mango, melons, red bell pepper, sweet potato, watercress, watermelon	057	Power Packed C
		077	Citrusberry
		185	Carotene Kick
		294	Pango Mango
Hypoglycemia	All fresh fruit and vegetable juice and fibre, cucumber, mango, seeds and their oils, yogurt	176	Grape & Green
		159	Cucumber Refresher
		298	Berry Mango
		306	Purple Rain
Indigestion	Cabbage, papaya, pineapple	030	Bellyful
		113	Gut Soother
		126	Digestaid
		359	Middle East Ginger

ailment	foods to eat	no.	juice title
Irritable bowel syndrome	All fruit and vegetable juice and fibre, all greens (such as broccoli, kale, parsley, spinach, watercress), bananas, cabbage, papaya, pineapple	172 113 254 285	Green Waldorf Gut Soother Papaya Pure Green Banana Creamy
Kidney problems	All greens (such as broccoli, kale, parsley, spinach, watercress), apricots, carrots, celery, cranberries, cucumber, melon, molasses, pears, pumpkin, red bell pepper, sweet potato, watermelon	105 210 162 167	Pink Pear II Pink Punch Water Water Everywhere Green Goddess
Memory problems	Fresh fruit and vegetable juices, especially berries, broccoli, citrus fruit, kale, kiwi fruit, watercress; seeds and their oils, wheatgerm	063 172 245	Orange Winter Crumble Green Waldorf Mango Blues Any smoothie with seeds/seed oil
Menopause-related problems	All fruit and vegetable juice and fibre, apples, celery, fennel, garlic, soy (soya), seeds and their oils, wheatgerm	012 069 209	Apple Cleanser Orange Aniseed Twist Crunch Morning Favourite Any smoothie with soy (soya) milk
Menstrual problems	All fruit and vegetable juice and fibre, beets, celery, fennel, garlic, seeds and their oils, soy (soya)	069 175 179	Orange Aniseed Twist Super Defender Beet Basic Any smoothie with soy (soya) milk
Motion sickness	Cabbage, carrots, ginger, peppermint	135 136 362 358	Carrot Crunch Carrot Digestif Mint & Honey Ginger Brew
Muscle cramps	All greens (such as broccoli, kale, parsley, spinach, watercress), molasses, seeds and their oils, wheatgerm	012 150 207 167	Apple Cleanser Chlorophyll Carrot Savoury Fruit Green Goddess
Obesity	All fruit and vegetable juice and fibre	019 133 209 248	Waldorf Salad Carrot Cleanser Crunch Morning Favourite Pineapple Zing
Osteoporosis prevention	All greens (such as broccoli, kale, parsley, spinach, watercress), garlic, milk, molasses, peaches, seeds and their oils, soy (soya) milk, yogurt	125 169 172 318	Green Pines Green 'n' Pear It Green Waldorf Peachy Passion
Premenstrual syndrome	All greens (such as broccoli, kale, parsley, spinach, watercress), celery, fennel, garlic, seeds and their oils, soy (soya)	067 169 172	Muddy Tonic Green 'n' Pear It Green Waldorf Any smoothie with soy (soya) milk
Prostate problems	Celery, fennel, fruit and vegetable fibre, garlic, molasses, soy (soya), seeds and their oils, tomatoes	188 203 172 283	Ginger Tom Tomorange Green Waldorf Creamy Black Banana

ailment	foods to eat	no.	juice title
Psoriasis	Apricots, broccoli, carrots, fruit and vegetable fibre, mango, pumpkin, red bell pepper, seeds and their oils, sweet potato, watercress	120 137 177 244	Ginger Zinger Carotene Catapult Creamy Green Nectargo
Shingles	Apricots, berries, broccoli, carrots, citrus fruit, garlic, kale, kiwi fruit, mango, melon, red bell pepper, sweet potato, seeds and their oils, watercress, watermelon	057 141 137 175	Power Packed C Cold War Carotene Catapult Super Defender
Sinusitis	Apricots, berries, broccoli, carrots, citrus fruit, kale, kiwi fruit, mango, melon, red bell pepper, sweet potato, seeds and their oils, watercress, watermelon	117 141 177 265	Black Pineapple Cold War Creamy Green Blue Healer
Sleeping problems	All greens (such as broccoli, kale, parsley, spinach, watercress), apples, bananas, milk, molasses, seeds, soy (soya) milk, yogurt	024 174 282 289	Apple Lullaby Green Lullaby Creamy Bananacot Banana Heaven
Sprains, strains & other injuries	All greens (such as broccoli, kale, parsley, spinach, watercress), garlic, milk, molasses, seeds and their oils, soy (soya) milk, yogurt	030 065 167 285	Bellyful Muddy Puddle Green Goddess Creamy Green Banana
Stomach ulcers	Cabbage, carrots, melon, papaya	030 136 173 254	Bellyful Carrot Digestif Sweet Green Melon Papaya Pure
Stress	All fruit and vegetable juice and fibre, all greens (such as broccoli, kale, parsley, spinach, watercress), berries, carrots, citrus fruit, milk, molasses, pineapple, red bell pepper, seeds and their oils, soy (soya) milk, wheatgerm, yogurt	133 172 285 315	Carrot Cleanser Green Waldorf Creamy Green Banana Pinkypine
Sunburn	Apricots, berries (especially blackcurrants), broccoli, carrots, citrus fruit, garlic, kiwi fruit, mango, pumpkin, red bell pepper, strawberries, sweet potatoes, watercress	062 002 277 279	Bitter Melon Apple Basic Creamy Cooler Green Sensation
Tonsillitis	Apricots, berries, broccoli, carrots, citrus fruit, garlic, kale, kiwi fruit, mango, melon, pineapple, red bell pepper, seeds and their oils, sweet potato, watercress, watermelon	117 116 141 265	Black Pineapple Pink Pineapple Cold War Blue Healer
Varicose veins	All fruit and vegetable juice and fibre, berries, broccoli, citrus fruit, kale, kiwi fruit, seeds and their oils, watercress, wheatgerm	002 055 082 320	Apple Basic Florida Blue Berry Bonanza Apricot Regular
Water retention	Celery, cucumber, melon, watermelon	206 161 213 162	Cool 'n' Pale II Mellow Melon Salty Sharp Melon Water Water Everywhere

Index

References are to page numbers, not recipes. This index should be used in conjunction with the index of ailments on pp.182–7 and the suggested juice courses on pp.176–8.